T'ai Chi Ch'uan

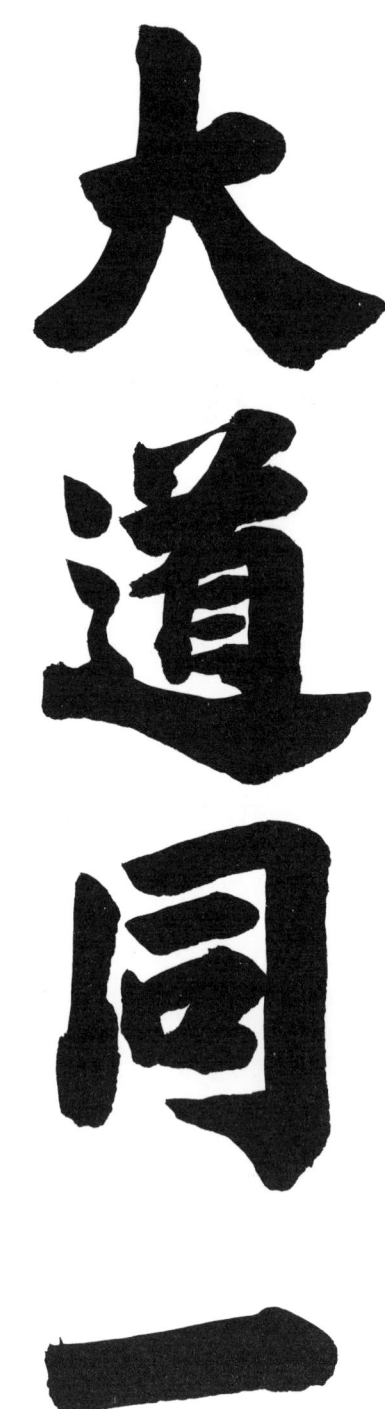

Becoming one with the Tao

T'ai Chi Ch'uan

Becoming One with the Tao

PETRA AND TOYO KOBAYASHI

TUTTLE PUBLISHING
Tokyo • Rutland, Vermont • Singapore

Please note that the publisher and authors of this instructional book are NOT RESPONSIBLE in any manner whatsoever for any injury that may result from practicing the techniques and/or following the instructions given within. Martial arts training can be dangerous—both to you and to others—if not practiced safely. If you're in doubt as to how to proceed or whether your practice is safe, consult with a trained martial arts teacher before beginning. Since the physical activities described herein may be too strenuous in nature for some readers, it is also essential that a physician be consulted prior to training.

Originally published as *T'ai Chi Ch'uan: Einswerden mit dem Tao,* by Heinrich Hugendubel Verlag.

English-language edition first published by Tuttle Publishing, an imprint of Periplus Editions (HK) Ltd., with editorial offices at 364 Innovation Drive, North Clarendon, Vermont 05759 U.S.A.

Copyright © 2006 Petra Kobayashi
Copyright © Heinrich Hugendubel Verlag, Kreuzlingen/München 1989
Alle Rechte vorbehalten.

All rights reserved. No part of this publication may be reproduced or utilized in any form or by any means, electronic or mechanical, including photocopying, recording, or by any information storage and retrieval system, without prior written permission from the publisher.

Translated and revised, 2006: Susan Rae Polzer and the author.

ISBN 10: 0-8048-3764-3
ISBN 13: 978-0-8048-3764-4

Library of Congress Cataloging-in-Publication Data
Kobayashi, Petra.
  T'ai chi ch'uan : becoming one with the Tao / Petra Kobayashi and Toyo Kobayashi.
      p. cm.
    Includes bibliographical references.
    ISBN 0-8048-3764-3 (pbk.)
  1. Tai chi. I. Kobayashi, Toyo. II. Title.
  GV504.K63 2008
  613.7'148—dc22   2006012840

Distributed by
North America, Latin America & Europe
Tuttle Publishing
364 Innovation Drive
North Clarendon, VT 05759-9436 U.S.A.
Tel: (1) 802 773-8930; Fax: (1) 802 773-6993
Email: info@tuttlepublishing.com
www.tuttlepublishing.com

Asia Pacific
Berkeley Books Pte. Ltd.
61 Tai Seng Avenue #02-12
Singapore 534167
Tel: (65) 6280-1330; Fax: (65) 6280-6290
Email: inquiries@periplus.com.sg
www.periplus.com

First edition
12 11 10 09 08   10 9 8 7 6 5 4 3 2

Printed in Singapore

TUTTLE PUBLISHING® is a registered trademark of Tuttle Publishing, a division of Periplus Editions (HK) Ltd.

CONTENTS

Acknowledgments	7
Foreword	9
Introduction	11
1. The Styles	18
Chen-Style	18
Yang-Style	19
Wu-Style	20
Sun-Style	20
Peking-Style	21
2. The Principles	23
3. Posture	25
4. How to Move	27
5. Relaxing	28
6. Exert No Force	29
7. Quotations from the Old Masters	30
8. Let Go (Release), Non-Action, and Follow	32
9. Sixty-Four Questions and Answers about T'ai Chi Ch'uan	33
10. Meditation	48
11. Energy	50
The Ch'i Development	50
Ch'i and Chin	51
12. Six Levels of Development	53
13. The Thirteen Basic Positions and the Techniques	55
14. The Song of the Thirteen Positions from Yang Cheng Fu	57
15. Advanced Practice	60
Sink	60
Center Equilibrium ("Centered Balance")	61
Full and Empty	62
Open and Close	63
16. Master Chi's Ten Important Rules for Advanced Practice	65
17. Two Aspects of the Forms: Practice and Application	66
18. Without Arms	67
19. Left Directs Left, Right Directs Right	68
20. The Bow Step	69

21. The Millstone Principle	70
22. The Millstone Exercise	72
23. Push Hands (Tui shou)	73
The Application of the Various Chin in Push Hands	74
Uprooting	74
Push Hands	76
24. The Short Form	80
25. Remarks about Practicing	81
26. Important Questions to Ask Yourself When Correcting Your Own Practice	86
27. Advice on Learning the Short Form	87
28. List of the Positions—Short Form	90
29. The Short Form	92
Glossary	185
Bibliography	187

ACKNOWLEDGMENTS

Our special thanks go to Swantje Autrum-Mulzer for the photographs; Master Lai Fung, Amsterdam, for the calligraphy; Peter Ebenhoch and V. Yelesejew for the drawings; Beatrix Schumacher, Janni Andriss, Jörg Lackner, and our daughters Ssu and Dhyana for their assistance; and Susan Rae Polzer for the English translation and help with the revision.

FOREWORD

T'ai Chi Ch'uan is an old Chinese-Taoist system of exercises whose history can be traced back to the T'ang Dynasty (A.D. 618–907). The basis of T'ai Chi Ch'uan are the classical treatises, texts from the old masters, in which the so-called principles[1] are written down. The most well-known exercise in T'ai Chi Ch'uan is the "form," a longer sequence of movements that is performed slowly, relaxed and flowing.

During the past centuries, T'ai Chi Ch'uan wasn't widespread in China. Only since the 1950s has it developed into a common sport and is increasingly well known in Southeast Asia as well as here in the West.

Since the principles permit variations in the exercises, T'ai Chi Ch'uan has continued to develop and change over the years. In this way, about ten main styles have evolved. Based on these foundations, simplified exercises have developed in almost incalculable variety, especially in recent years. However, the refined adjustments of the principles were often lost along the way.

One reason for the wide popularity of T'ai Chi Ch'uan lies, without a doubt, in the manifold possibilities of its application. T'ai Chi Ch'uan is not only a holistic health exercise, physiotherapy, relaxation and breathing exercise; it also guides the human being on the path that leads to spiritual realization (harmony with the Tao) and makes effective self-defense possible.

If one practices T'ai Chi Ch'uan solely for health reasons, then one can profit from many directions in T'ai Chi. Experience shows that many positive health results come from simply practicing the fundamental principles, such as soft, relaxed, gentle, and flowing. However, if one wants to become more intensely involved, one should turn to a T'ai Chi[2] that contains the refinement that distinguishes the original T'ai Chi Ch'uan.

Both of the first styles to become known in T'ai Chi Ch'uan, the Chen-style and the Yang-style that developed out of it, can be helpful here as orientation. The common origin of nearly all known T'ai Chi Ch'uan directions today exist in their forms. Valuable information about T'ai Chi Ch'uan in the Yang-style is offered in books and texts from its last important masters: Yang Cheng-Fu, Cheng Man-Ch'ing, Chen Wei Ming, and Tung Ying Chieh. Their works (see bibliography), which have only recently been translated into Western languages, describe the little-known art of advanced T'ai Chi Ch'uan. In addition to the classical treatises, they contribute to the classical T'ai Chi literature.

The teachers named emphatically point out that, without a refined form and practice of the exercises based on the principles, a perfection in the sense of T'ai Chi Ch'uan can't be achieved.

In the book presented here, the foundations for a refined practice are imparted as they have been passed down in the Yang-style. As is the nature of the thing, a deeper understanding of many parts of the contents and their connections to each other only become obvious when they have been confirmed by personal experience.

---

1 The characteristics of the structure and practice of the exercises are determined by the principles.
2 T'ai Chi is the common abbreviation for T'ai Chi Ch'uan.

In the practical part of this book, we describe the short form of the Yang-style (three parts) in the tradition of Professor Cheng Man-Ch'ing, which we learned from one of his main students, Dr. Chi Chiang Tao. In addition, a basic partner exercise (Push Hands) is included. The short form of Cheng Man-Ch'ing belongs to the most widely known exercises in T'ai Chi, and it has especially found many followers in the West. It is based upon the long form of Yang Ch'eng Fu, who was the teacher of Cheng Man-Ch'ing.

For its English-language publication, this book has been carefully revised. Almost twenty years have passed since its completion and initial publication in Germany! After Dr. Chi retired from teaching in 1989, we worked on his advice with Liu Si-Heng in Taipeh, Taiwan who continued the school of Cheng Man-Ch'ing there. When private travel was allowed in the People's Republic of China in the early nineties, we used this opportunity to further advance our study of T'ai Chi with well-known teachers of the Yang-style. Among others, we studied with Fu Zhong Wen in Shanghai, and Ma Chang Xun, Shi Ming, and Zhang Guojian in Peking. With increased experience, it became clear to us that much of what we had learned about the inner energetic aspect of T'ai Chi could be excellently combined with the short form as we learned it from Dr. Chi. This means that such information has also contributed to this revision, at least in the approach.

A growing interest has been noticed in many practitioners to delve deeper into the spirit of T'ai Chi Ch'uan and to arrive at a more effective way of practicing. This book would like to be an orientation and help for those who are so inclined.

Petra Kobayashi

INTRODUCTION

T'ai Chi Ch'uan—an Exercise to Maintain Health and to Prevent Illness[3] *by DR. CHI CHIANG TAO*

T'ai Chi Ch'uan is a Chinese exercise system from ancient times that serves to maintain good health, to heal illnesses, to support self-defense and physical and mental recuperation. The number of practitioners is growing daily. If one goes early in the morning to a quiet place in the New Park of Taipeh or if one walks along the shore of the Tam Chih river where the air is fresher than in the city, one sees groups of people, usually middle to older aged, practicing T'ai Chi Ch'uan with focused attention and a relaxed posture. This type of physical exercise is not only favored by us but is also practiced in Chinese communities abroad. I have heard that in the headquarters of the United Nations they have also organized a T'ai Chi club where qualified teachers of this skill give instruction. Last year the T'ai Chi enthusiasts of Taiwan invited all the outstanding T'ai Chi specialists in the country to form a committee for the study of this method and to join the American-Chinese cultural and business association. Members of the committee meet each Sunday morning to study the practice and application of this method.

Why do so many people, Chinese as well as foreigners, devote so much enthusiasm to T'ai Chi Ch'uan?

Some of the reasons for this are:

1. The complete sequence of the T'ai Chi Ch'uan movements, which have many positive effects, needs only about fifteen minutes; a shortened form only five to six minutes to perform.

2. A small space is sufficient to practice T'ai Chi Ch'uan.

3. In many other physical exercises, so much force is used that the practitioner is exhausted at the end. In T'ai Chi Ch'uan, however, one learns to use as little force as possible, and one feels refreshed and also mentally alert rather than tired after practicing.

4. T'ai Chi Ch'uan can heal many illnesses.

T'ai Chi Ch'uan and Medical Epistemology

Modern medicine considers physical exercise to be a good method to cure sickness. In the past, one believed that physical exercises weren't appropriate for heart problems, for example.

Today, influential doctors suggest that even patients with heart problems should pursue moderate physical exercise. They have acknowledged that exercising is a good

---

[3] This article by Dr. Chi appeared in 1965 in the Taiwanese magazine *West and East Monthly* (shortened here and newly translated from German, 2004).

method of preventing heart problems. Dr. White, who treated past President Eisenhower for his heart problems, said: "In order to maintain a healthy heart, a certain amount of exercise is necessary. Appropriate exercise can lengthen a life since not only the strength of the heart functions but also the elasticity of the muscles, the interaction of the nerves and the breathing movement are decisive parts in the creation of good circulation."

British doctors have conducted a large-scale investigation that shows that people who work in offices and don't regularly participate in physical exercises have a heart attack more frequently.

Dr. Hoffmann, royal doctor for the Prince of Prussia, said: "Exercise is the best medicine for human beings. Its effect on human health is incredible."

In China, the famous surgeon Hua To developed the five animal exercises during the late Han Dynasty.[4] They were based on the primary movements of the tiger, the bear, the monkey, the stag, and the bird. He said: "Movement helps the digestion and the circulation so that illnesses can be prevented."

If exercise is so important for good health, in what form should it be created to bring about the best possible results? Dr. Hsueh Yu-hsing, chief of staff for geriatric illnesses at the Veterans General Hospital in Taiwan writes: "When a person becomes old, his bones become fragile. Exhausting and difficult exercises should, therefore, be avoided. T'ai Chi Ch'uan is one of the best exercises for older people. It helps against many complaints, is good against rheumatism, heart problems and high blood pressure."

T'ai Chi Ch'uan is different from the well-known ball games, exercises on or with equipment, and the usual gymnastics. Most of these exercises limit themselves to one-sided body movement and don't proceed in harmony with natural breathing. With them, there is an acceleration of the pulse rate, intensive breathing, and often heavy perspiration. With T'ai Chi Ch'uan, on the other hand, a coordination of all the body parts occurs in the movement. Its relaxed and round movements use the joints evenly. When T'ai Chi Ch'uan is practiced long enough, it leads to a recovery of the tonicity and the elasticity of the bones and the joints as well as to a strengthening of the blood vessels. Even the blood vessels that have lost their elasticity can gradually regenerate. It is also a good exercise for the central nervous system so that neurasthenia (weak nerves) and insomnia can be cured.

Many friends who practice T'ai Chi Ch'uan tell me that T'ai Chi Ch'uan has been an unexpected remedy for a variety of illnesses such as allergic colds, diabetes, and tuberculosis of the lungs.

According to modern medical investigations, many illnesses develop from nervous tension (stress) or are caused by emotional suffering. In the investigations of Dr. Chang Hsueh-hsien from the National Taiwan University Hospital, it became obvious that nervous tension in animals reduces the resistance to bacteria and viruses. He writes: "When animal cells are attacked by a virus, they produce a substance that surrounds the cell to protect it. If the energy of this substance is stronger than the virus, no illness results. When the animal, however, is stressed-out, a large amount of hormones are poured into the body. These influence the production of the above-mentioned substance and therein, the resistance of the animal."

---

4 Han Dynasty (205 B.C. – A.D. 220)

Dr. Hans Selye, an American specialist for glandular illnesses, warned people who follow a high-stress lifestyle: "When a person is very tense, he can be poisoned from the hormones that his own body produces against this tension. This type of poisoning can have a worse effect than alcohol poisoning, for example."

Dr. Joseph Kennedy, former Marine doctor, writes in his book, *Relax and Live:* "The results of nervous tension are insomnia and a shortened life. When one knows how to relax, one can lengthen one's life."

Practicing T'ai Chi Ch'uan with its harmonious movements and the emphasis on relaxation can help one to be more relaxed even in our modern industrial society today, with strenuous office work and in overfilled transportation, subjected to the noises of a large city.

T'ai Chi Ch'uan for the Elderly

The rapid advancement in medical science and the improvement of the health systems have contributed to almost eliminating many illnesses such as malaria, typhoid, and cholera. Also lung tuberculosis can now often be cured. In this way, the average life expectancy has been extended. With the increase in the number of older people, however, there are also more problems with illnesses of the elderly. At the moment, older people in Taiwan comprise 5 percent of the total population; in the European countries and in North America it is already 20 percent. When a person ages, his physical and mental functions tend to slow down and deteriorate. Frequent illnesses of the aged are chronic bronchitis; arteriosclerosis, or hardening of the arteries; heart problems; malignant nodes; insomnia; arthritis; rheumatoid arthritis, and diabetes. Briefly stated, the illnesses from which an older person suffers are essentially the results of physiological changes with a chronic deterioration of the general condition.

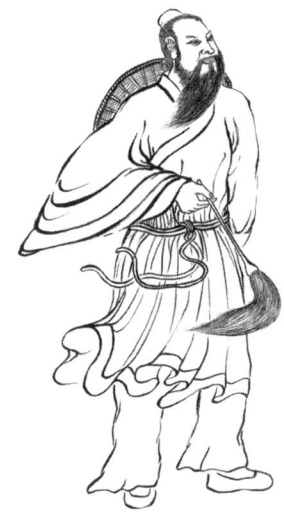

*Chang San-Feng,
the legendary founder
of T'ai Chi Ch'uan*

A remedy for the elderly isn't as easy to find as for those in younger years. Frequently several illnesses appear at the same time. The gradual decline of the liver and kidney functions hampers the elimination of medicines taken and leads to a poisoning of the body. When T'ai Chi Ch'uan is practiced regularly over an extended period of time, the functions of the entire body are strengthened.

As a result, senility is counteracted. An example of this is: when we practice T'ai Chi Ch'uan in a group, we can observe how a seventy-year-old performs partner exercises with a younger person. His flexibility, sensitivity, and mental awareness are no different than that of the younger people.

Important Points for the Practice of T'ai Chi Ch'uan

T'ai Chi Ch'uan is an exceptionally comprehensive physical exercise that is defined by numerous rules. Therefore, it is said that: "T'ai Chi Ch'uan is easy to learn but difficult to perform masterfully," and "ten years of practice is not enough for a public performance."

When one wants to learn T'ai Chi Ch'uan as an exercise for one's health and practices two or three hours a week for several months, one can learn the short form; the long form requires twice the time. After one has received correction over a longer period of time, one is capable of practicing according to the rules. If one wants to master the exercises for practical purposes, however, the length of time one needs to show progress is determined by various factors such as intellectual grasp, teaching methods, and the efforts of the student. My opinion is that it is better to begin under the personal guidance of a teacher. Of course, one can also learn T'ai Chi Ch'uan from books; however, the accuracy of the performance leaves something to be desired, one can easily become accustomed to small mistakes.

Independent from the reason why T'ai Chi Ch'uan is practiced, it is first and foremost important to keep the movements light, lively, balanced, and slow and to perform them with as little force as possible. The body is erect and relaxed, the buttocks hang loose, the rib cage (thorax) is somewhat lowered (but not caved in), the head should be held upright, and the eyes look straight ahead. An old T'ai Chi Ch'uan aphorism says: "When the head hangs down and the leg position leaves something to be desired, someone didn't receive the correct instruction."

Every movement should come from the *Tan T'ien*. (Tan T'ien is a Taoist expression, which literally means, "the field for the planting of the Tan," a substance that according to the Taoist teachings confers upon the owner immortality and supernatural strengths. The position of the Tan T'ien in a person of average height can be determined in the following manner: 3–4 cm. (1.2–1.5 inches) under the naval, one divides an imaginary horizontal line reaching to the spine into three parts. The Tan T'ien is then located two thirds of the way to the spine.)

All the movements follow the unity of the body. When moving forward, the heel touches the floor first; when moving backward, it is the toes. In all the movements, the center of gravity remains stable so that the body doesn't lose balance. All the movements flow into each other without a pause. The following significant words should always accompany the practitioner: "upright, relaxed, continuous, and balanced."

Inhaling and exhaling should occur through the nose, not through the mouth. The air that is breathed in and out through the nose should have a fine and continuous flow; at the same time, the breathing should not be externally noticeable. When the breath flows regularly, lightly, slowly, and deeply, then one has attained the level of natural breathing.

When one stretches the arms out, one should breathe out, and when one pulls the arms inward, one should breathe in. When the body is raised, breathe in; when it moves down, breathe out. During the turns, one breathes the way that occurs naturally. An additional important point is the adjustment of the practice to the physical condition. For an ill and fragile person, one can't set the same expectations as for a healthy person.

Rules to Be Observed before and after Practicing

An open place in the fresh air is best suited for the practice of T'ai Chi Ch'uan. If such a place is not available, one can also practice at home. When possible, one should open a window. One shouldn't practice directly after a large meal. After practicing, it is advisable to walk back and forth a bit. In the first months of practicing, it can sometimes happen that one feels a weakening of one's strength, tiredness and a resistance against practicing. This doesn't need to make one uneasy. This period is called, "the transition of growing strength." When it is overcome, one will discover improvements in one's practicing.

Important Points for Use in Self-Defense

T'ai Chi Ch'uan is not only for health and personal development but also for self-defense. The efficiency of T'ai Chi Ch'uan for self-defense is often questioned by outsiders. The gentle and slowly executed movements hardly appear to be appropriate for self-defense. I shall, therefore, explain some aspects of self-defense; the principle exercise for learning self-defense is *Tui shou* (Push Hands). Tui shou is the name for a partner exercise in which the basic movements practiced are *"Peng"* (Ward-Off), *"Lu"* (Rollback), *"Chi"* (Press), and *"An"* (Push).

The first step in learning Push Hands is the uniform movement of the hips and legs as well as the indication of the movement intended by the opponent, named *Ting Chin*. Ting Chin is a technical expression, literally meaning, "Listen to the strength of the opponent." It is equivalent to the *Chi Chin*, which means "to sense force."

In Push Hands, hard muscle strength should be completely eliminated; one should be calm and composed and attempt to follow the movements of one's opponent. If he pushes me in a particular direction, I concentrate my attention on this direction. I follow him in his movements with continuous *"Chan"* (sticking and lifting), *"Lien"* (connecting), *"Tieh"* (horizontal sticking) and *"Sui"* (sticking from behind). After extensive practicing of Push Hands, the sensitivity is so well developed that the "extra weight of a feather is felt" and that "a fly can't land on the body without bringing it into movement," as they say in the classical texts.

When, in a duel, Mr. A. wants to push Mr. B. away, he must, for example, bring his hand, his wrist, his elbow, or his shoulder in contact with Mr. B. This is called "contact force." When B. feels the contact force from A., he pulls his body away immediately and while doing so, goes into a slight crouch (relax and sink). In T'ai Chi Ch'uan, this is called, *"Tsou hua,"* which means, "the transformation of the approaching force through a withdrawal movement." Although A. places a lot of force into his thrust, the impact on B.'s body would be prevented by the use of Tsou hua because the approaching force would find no point of attack. In that way, it would be a strike into a vacuum. At the same time, when A. loses his balance, B. can pull him with minimal strength and would surely make him fall down. The classical texts speak in this connection of the "trigger release strength of 4 ounces (about 100 g), that can divert the impact of a thousand pounds and can transform it into an equivalent return."

In a treatise about T'ai Chi Ch'uan it says: "In T'ai Chi Ch'uan, movement is overcome by calmness (non-action) and rigidity conquered by flexibility." All these principles are important in T'ai Chi Ch'uan. Yang Cheng-Fu, the teacher of my teacher, says: "The Tsou-hua method is similar to pushing away a bottle gourd that is swimming in water and that offers no resistance upon which force can be used." The desire to conquer a master of T'ai Chi Ch'uan through hard muscle force is like an attempt to catch the wind or a shadow.

In the Tsou-hua method, so-called tenacious energy is applied. It is different in its effectiveness, therefore, from the evasive actions applied in many martial arts.

When we are attacked by an opponent, we only follow the principles determined by the exercises but use no force. In Tui shou, which literally means "push hands" or "shove," it isn't the force of the hands that is important but rather the impact of the tenacious energy that originates in the uniform movement of the legs and the hips. The application of tenacious energy can be compared to the shooting of an arrow, where the bowstring must first be drawn. The technical term in T'ai Chi Ch'uan for this is *"Fa Fong"* (discharge).

Highly trained practitioners in the Yang school can hurl their opponent many meters away without using force. Such a high level of perfection in T'ai Chi Ch'uan, however, can only be achieved with great effort. The advanced art of T'ai Chi Ch'uan will disappear when no one is prepared to devote himself so intensely.

Final Remarks

When the practitioner is more advanced, his interest in T'ai Chi Ch'uan will be heightened through practicing Push Hands. Just like the form, Push Hands is even a good method for use against mental illness. The health of people who have encountered difficult strokes of fate or suffer suppressed problems is often damaged. Practice can be of help because it develops harmony and inner strength in the individual.

After the basic exercises of the T'ai Chi Ch'uan (form and Tui shou), one can learn *Ta Lu*. Ta Lu, the "large pull" or the "large rollback" is the technical term for an exercise where two partners perform the basic movements of *"Tsai"* (pull), *"Lieh"* (divide), *"Chou"* (elbow strike), and *"Kao"* (shoulder push).

In addition to these exercises, the T'ai Chi sword form is the best known. The same rules apply here as in the other forms. The T'ai Chi sword form is also an excellent method of physical and mental recuperation.

On the basis of the unquestionably extensive advantages of T'ai Chi Ch'uan, every practitioner will greatly profit from practicing. T'ai Chi Ch'uan is recommended for people of all age groups.

1. The Styles

In the following section, the most well-known of the ten main styles of T'ai Chi Ch'uan—the Chen-, Yang-, Sun-, Wu-, and Peking-styles—will be briefly described. They represent different combination possibilities of the exercises. Their forms differ from each other through, among other things, changing the placement of the arms and the legs within the framework of the principles as well as various sequences of the positions.

Chen-Style

The oldest known style of T'ai Chi Ch'uan is the Chen-style.[5] There are two main theories about its origin. One of them says that the founder of the Chen-style, Chen Wang-Ting (1597–1664),[6] had T'ai Chi Ch'uan passed down to him from Wang Tsung-Yueh from the Ming dynasty (1368–1644).

According to the other version, Chen Wang-Ting developed the Chen-style himself from the basis of the well-known book *Ch'uan Chin* and his own knowledge of Taoist meditation practices.[7]

Exceptional masters of the Chen-style after Chen Wang-Ting were Chen So Kao, Chen Ching Po, and Chen Chang-Hsiang (1771–1853).

Until Chen Chang-Hsiang, the Chen-style was only handed down within the extended Chen family. He was the first to instruct an outsider, Yang Lu-Ch'an, the founder of the Yang-style.

Well-known masters of the Chen-style after Chen Chang-Hsiang were Chen Yi-Hsi and his son, Chen Fa-Ku (1887–1957). It is said about Chen Fa-Ku that his *Ch'i* (inner energy) was so strongly developed that window shutters and roof shingles rattled when he practiced. He taught in Peking and had many students.

There are three main directions within the Chen-style:

1. Old style

2. New style

3. Small style

1. The "old style" refers back to Chen Chang-Hsiang. It is practiced with deeply bent knees. The arms and legs depict large circular arches. The "old style" contains a series of

---

[5] The styles are generally named after the founder.

[6] The transcription used here is commonly found in English language T'ai Chi literature. It is derived from the earlier official language, Cantonese, and is used by expatriate Chinese in Southeast Asia and Taiwan and often in the West. The Pinjin transcription, which is promoted by the present Chinese government, developed from the Han Chinese. T'ai Chi Ch'uan is called Taijiquan, Tao is called Dao, I Ching (I Ging) is called Yiying, Chi Kung is called Qigonq, and so on.

[7] Chi Che-Kwong (1529–1587). See Huang, *The Fundamentals of T'ai Chi Ch'uan,* page 48. Please note: the pages listed here referring to other publications are based upon editions that were available in 1989, when the German version of this book was first published.

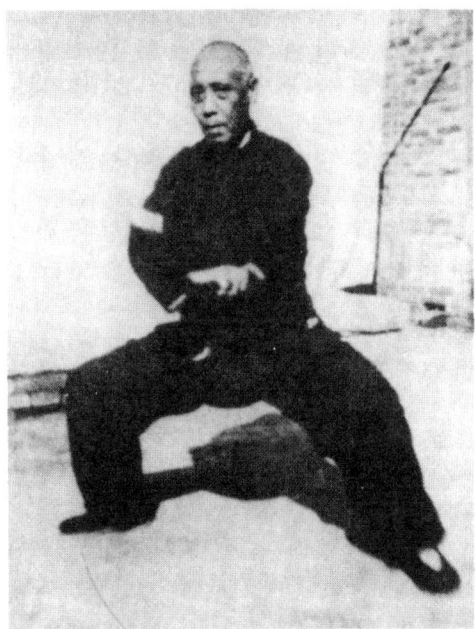
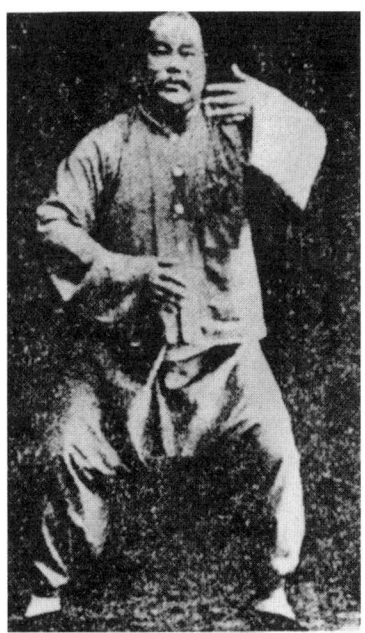

Chen Fa-Ku *Yang Cheng-Fu*

difficult to perform motions, such as high jumps. The speed is usually a steady slowness; exceptions, in addition to the jumps, are the fist and feet thrusts. These are emphasized and performed rapidly.

2. The new style refers back to Chen Yu Pen. He simplified many of the complicated motions of the old style.

3. The small style was developed by Cheng Ch'ing P'ing, who studied with Chen Yu Pen. Economical movements are characteristic of the small style. It is practiced relatively fast.

Yang-Style

Yang Lu-Ch'an (1799–1872) developed the Yang-style, which is named after his given name, Yang, which means "the unsurpassable." His family name was actually Yeung. The spread of T'ai Chi Ch'uan is especially attributed to him. He wanted to make T'ai Chi Ch'uan available to many people. Through his public teaching, he broke with the old tradition in which martial arts, meditation practices, and often also exercises for health were only passed on to a small, select circle of students or within the family.[8] Following his example, the masters of the Chen-style also began to make their knowledge available.

Yang Lu-Ch'an's form has not been handed down. Both his sons, Yang Pan-Hou (1837–1892) and Yang Chien-Hu (1839–1917), changed his form.

Yang Chien-Hu is said to have reduced the size of the movements. Yang Pan-Hou, however, is said to have practiced with wide-reaching movements. Yang Chien-Hu's son, Yang Cheng-Fu, was the first to put together the so-called "traditional form" of the

---

[8] Matsuda. *Secret of Chin-jia-chi*, page 23 (only available in a Japanese edition).

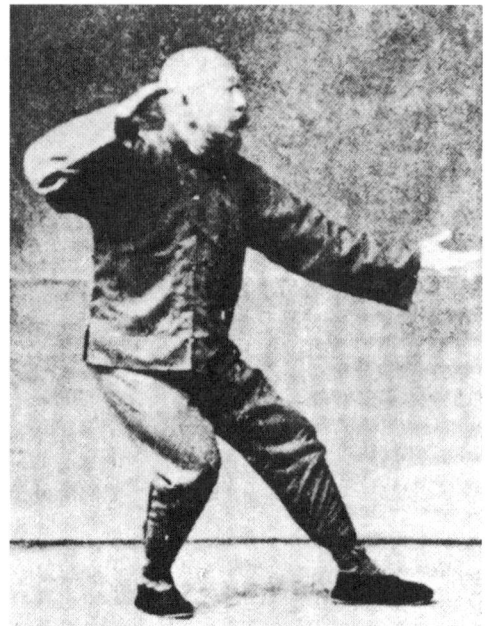 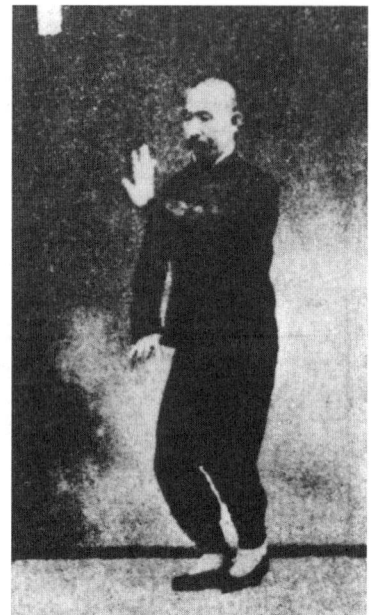

Chen Wei-Ming *Sun Lu-Tang*

Yang-style. It has been handed down through photographs and drawings; most of today's Yang-style forms are taken from Yang Cheng-Fu's long form. His student, Cheng Man-Ch'ing (1900–1975), developed the short form of the Yang-style from the long form of his teacher (see page 80). His comparatively easy-to-learn short form has contributed considerably to the spread of T'ai Chi in modern times.

Wu-Style

Wu Ch'ien-Ch'uan (1870–1942) is considered the founder of Wu-style, which is named after him. But his father, Wu Quan-You (1834–1902), who studied with Yang Pan Hou, also played an important role in the development of the Wu-style. Wu Ch'ien-Ch'uan taught in Shanghai. The Wu-style is still widely known in Shanghai and the surrounding area.

Sun-Style

The Sun-style refers back to Sun Lu-Tang (1861–1932). Sun Lu-Tang began to study T'ai Chi Ch'uan at the age of fifty years. Before that, he had learned Hsing I from Li Kuei-Yuan and Kuo Yun-Shen, as well as Pa Kua from Ch'eng Ting-Hua. His T'ai Chi teacher was Hoa Wei-Chin (1849–1920, Hoa-style).

Sun Lu-Tang is the author of several books about Hsing I, Pa Kua, and T'ai Chi Ch'uan. Elements of Hsing I and Pa Kua have slipped into Sun-style. In comparison to the Yang-style, it is practiced with the knees less bent.

Sun Lu-Tang's daughter, Sun Jian-Yun, belongs to his outstanding students. The Sun-style has found little dissemination.

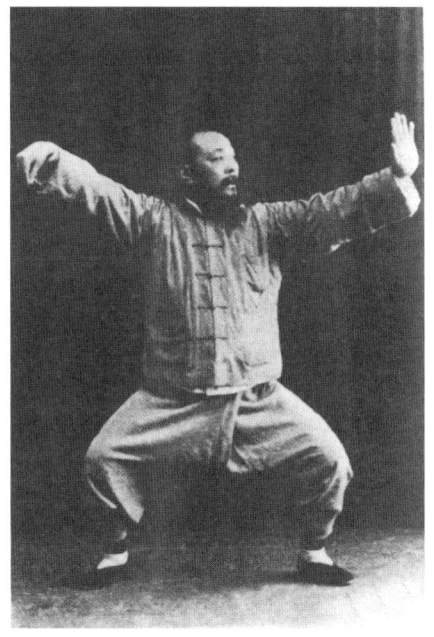 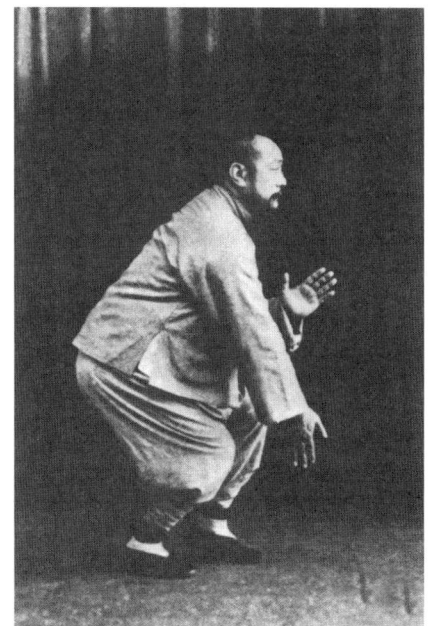

Wu Ch-ien-Chu'an

Peking-Style

Peking-style was essentially compiled by Li T'ien-Yi based on Yang Cheng-Fu's long form. Insight into its emergence came with the publication of the first T'ai Chi book after the Chinese Cultural Revolution.[9] In the foreword of this book it says, among other things:

T'ai Chi Ch'uan, one of the greatest Chinese cultural treasures, is resurrected again through Mao Tse Tung's support. He has emphasized the importance of athletic exercises, including T'ai Chi Ch'uan. In this way, T'ai Chi Ch'uan became a public sport. In 1956, in order to make the practicing of T'ai Chi Ch'uan available for many people, the Peking-style was put together as simplified exercises based on the traditional T'ai Chi Ch'uan. In 1958, partner exercises, a long form and T'ai Chi sword were also made available to the public. To satisfy the great interest of many people, this book now appears to assist in practicing.[10]

The old styles—Chen, Yang, Wu, and Sun—still exist, in spite of the temporary repression of T'ai Chi Ch'uan during the Cultural Revolution. Today, the Peking-style is the most widespread style in the People's Republic of China.

---

9 A publication of the National Sport Association, People's Republic of China, 1962.
10 The area of meditative-spiritual T'ai Chi Ch'uan and its Taoist background is usually not mentioned in the official Chinese publications. Until recently, new editions of old Chinese T'ai Chi books had only appeared in Hong Kong and Taiwan.

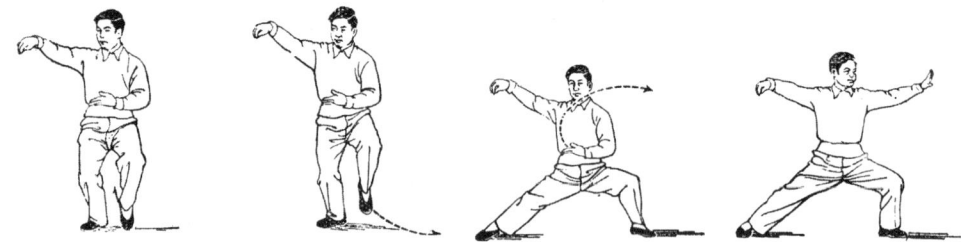

Chen-style

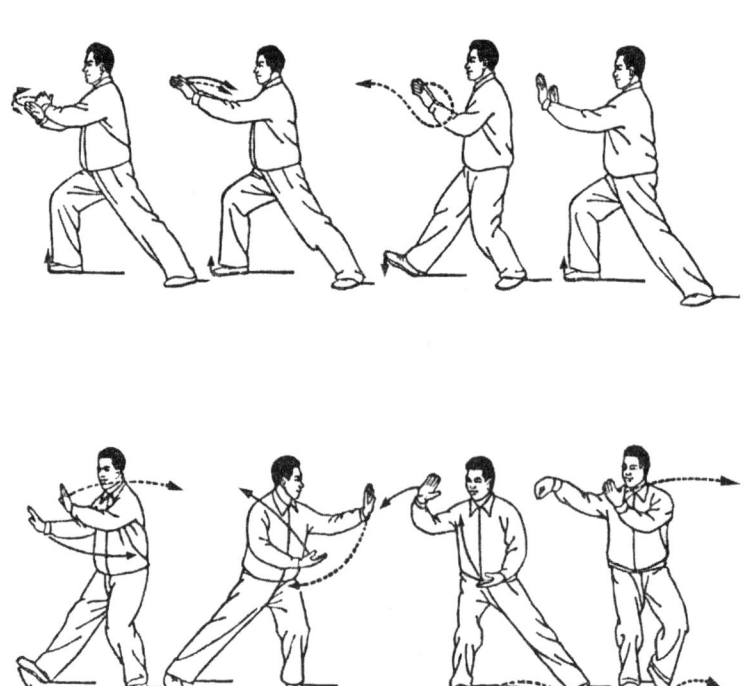

Peking-style

2. The Principles

The principles are the heart of T'ai Chi Ch'uan as it has been handed down over the centuries. They are written down in the classical treatises and other texts by the old masters.[11] In very short, memorable sentences, they establish the shape and performance of T'ai Chi Ch'uan and convey the philosophical-theoretical foundations of the exercises.

The principles mirror the long experience in Chinese society with exercises for health, martial arts, and meditation practices that were in full bloom long before the development of T'ai Chi Ch'uan. Observing them in their entirety, the Taoist background of T'ai Chi Ch'uan becomes especially clear.

Here are some examples:

1. In the principles that determine the structure of the movements and the method of energy development, the practical application of the Taoist philosophy of Yin and Yang can be followed in detail—as for example, in the constant changing of the movement from full (*Yang*) to empty (*Yin*) and the many reciprocal movements.

2. Principles that effect the way of movement and mental attitude, as in release (let go), yield, follow, and withdraw, have their equivalents in Taoist philosophy.

3. The uppermost rule in Taoist exercises, the orientation on the nature of human beings, also applies in T'ai Chi. It claims to be true to this maxim through its "natural way" in an especially complete manner. Knowledge about the existing conditions of the physical body and the subtle energy realm (see page 48) has come to be used in the principles in such a way that the best possible natural state is through their realization.

In the thirteen basic positions (see page 55), the first sequences of movements to be handed down in T'ai Chi Ch'uan, the principles have taken on form, so to speak. Within them, the three main aspects of T'ai Chi Ch'uan—health, self-defense, and meditation—come equally into play. The movement sequences contained in the thirteen basic positions are based upon techniques for self-defense. At the same time, they guarantee the optimal effects on the state of health and create, moreover, the best prerequisites for meditative practice in the T'ai Chi Ch'uan sense.[12]

The detailed description of the fundamental principles is one of the priorities of this book. Following is a brief version of the most important principles.

---

[11] See glossary.
[12] For a description of the effect of T'ai Chi Ch'uan on physical and mental-spiritual health, see *Der Weg des T'ai Chi Ch'uan,* currently available only in German.

Important Principles of T'ai Chi Ch'uan

---

upright - balanced - continuous - slow
unified - soft - gentle - light - rounded
lively

*

let go (release) - relax - yield
follow - sink - root
straighten from within
full and empty - open and close

*

no arms - no force
"Millstone" movement - coordinated movement
natural breathing - meditative state of mind

---

3. Posture

The posture is described in the classical texts. It should be upright, comfortable, and natural. The spine should thereby be held "as if one had swallowed a pole."

In this position of the spine, the torso doesn't need to be held in an unnatural way by the ligaments. This provides the best possible conditions for the perpendicular effect of the force of gravity with which the sinking of Ch'i and all the attached developments are connected.

Practicing in a natural, upright posture occurs logically from the alignment of T'ai Chi Ch'uan with human nature. The aspired erect position of the spine here must appear—if one goes from the S-form curvature of the spinal column—as unnatural and, therefore, even in the opposing direction to the T'ai Chi Ch'uan path.[13] The upright position of the spinal column is, however, one of the basic principles of T'ai Chi Ch'uan. Like all other principles, this is also consistent with experience. The meaning and the implication of this position is then experienced latest when the perception of Ch'i occurs. Yang Cheng-Fu said: "If the back is held upright, the energy can flow in an incomparable manner."

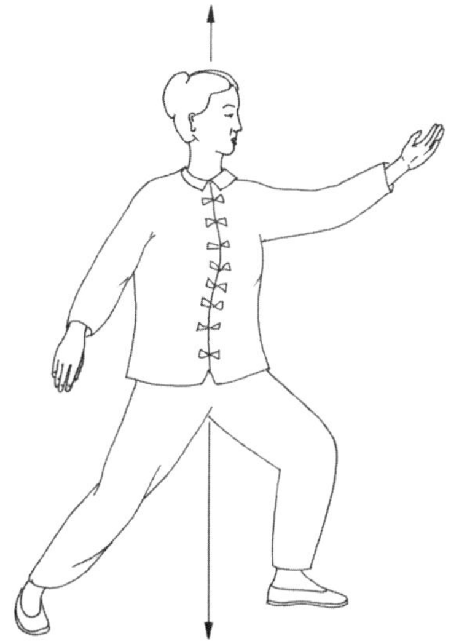

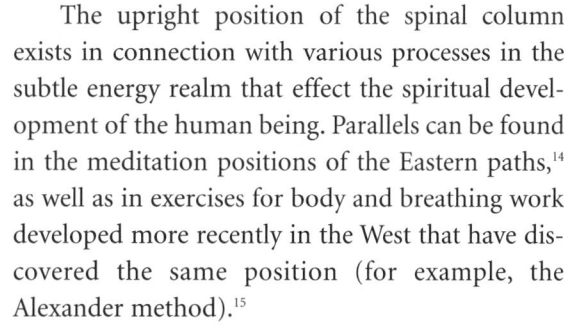

The upright position of the spinal column exists in connection with various processes in the subtle energy realm that effect the spiritual development of the human being. Parallels can be found in the meditation positions of the Eastern paths,[14] as well as in exercises for body and breathing work developed more recently in the West that have discovered the same position (for example, the Alexander method).[15]

The correct performance of many principles—such as full and empty; right directs right, left directs left; millstone; let go (release); sink; and straighten from within—can't be achieved without the erect position of the spinal column.

Since posture is of such essential meaning in T'ai Chi Ch'uan, it is assumed that the practitioners correct their posture themselves and work on it. Even minimal approaches to the ideal posture are beneficial to the developments in the subtle energy realm. Unfortunately posture frequently doesn't receive the necessary attention. In many T'ai Chi directions, the awareness of it is often lost.

---

13 In self-defense it also appears that the erect position of the spine is not beneficial but apparently rather limits our possibilities to react. Skillful T'ai Chi Ch'uan, however, is precisely characterized by the ability to meet attacks in this position.

14 Zen Master, Gesshin Prahasaddharma-Roshi: "Posture means to manifest the Buddha."

15 A more exact description of these relationships can be read in *Weg des T'ai Chi Ch'uan*, pages 31–38. This book is currently available only in German.

Cheng Man-Ch'ing refers specifically to this handed-down position in T'ai Chi Ch'uan. It can be found in the same way in the exceptional masters of the Chen-style (for example, Chen Fa-Kua). Dr. Chi assured us that in the Yang Pan Hou tradition, which goes back to Yang Lu Ch'an, the upright straight posture was practiced in the same way.

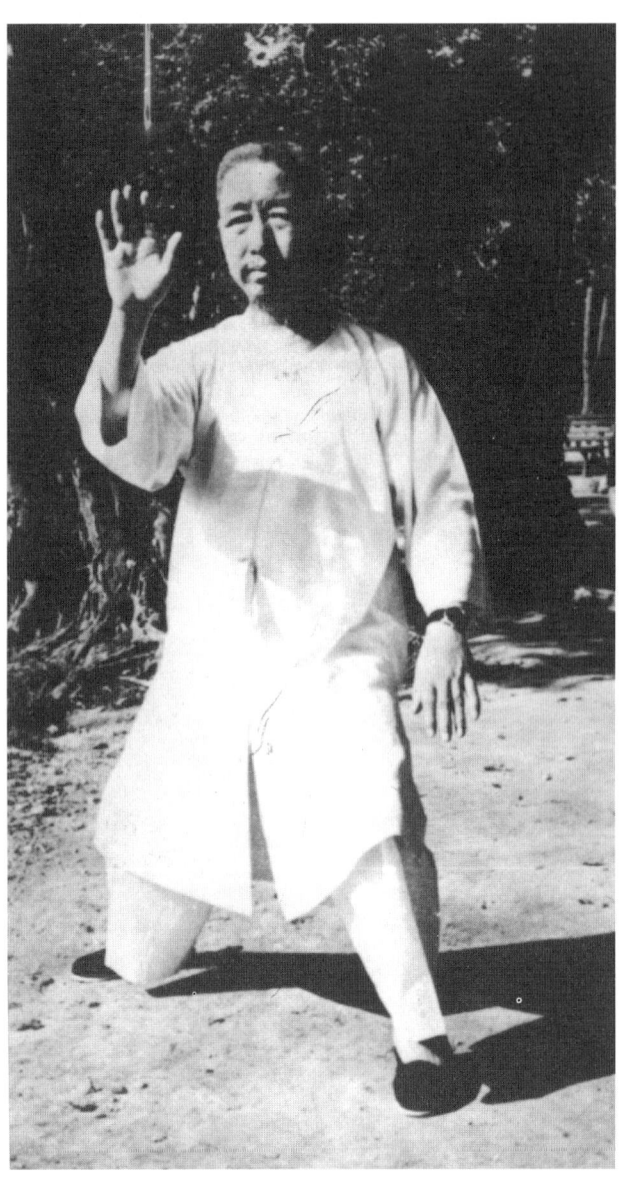

Cheng Man-Ch'ing

4. How to Move

The way to move is not only relaxed, natural, light, and lively but also embedded in a definite pace. In the classical treatises, this is compared with pulling a silk thread from a cocoon: "Pull it too rapidly, it breaks; pull it too slowly, it doesn't unwind." Experience shows that one must acquire the correct way of moving through attentive practicing. It can only be accomplished in the spirit of T'ai Chi Ch'uan when the principles such as sink, straighten from within, center equilibrium, full and empty, as well as open and close[16] are correctly applied and lead to a polarization in the movement. With increasing Ch'i development through the activation of energy, the movement then occurs as if by itself and can be performed lightly, naturally, and in a lively way with the least possible effort. This kind of movement is in harmony with Taoist values.

Other ways of moving disseminated by T'ai Chi Ch'uan don't agree with the principles to the same extent; for example, the "made" movement that lacks letting go and naturalness and the too slow one that can't bring the Ch'i to flow. Also, the widespread only gentle and relaxed way of moving shows no real liveliness because the polarization is missing.

---
16 See page 63.

5. Relaxing

Relaxed movement is characteristic for T'ai Chi Ch'uan. This is true regardless of whether the limbs of the body are raised or lowered, or whether we move forward or backward.

Practicing relaxation while moving is an important aspect of T'ai Chi Ch'uan. Relaxation in a quiet position is relatively easy to achieve and has many positive effects. When we move out of a quiet position, however, we tend to fall back into our frequently tense way of moving. Since we spend a large part of the day in movement, T'ai Chi Ch'uan helps us to be relaxed in our daily life, too.

It is often assumed that we are already in a relaxed condition after practicing for a short period. Long-standing tension, which usually comes from decades of incorrect posture and the associated bad habits in movement, can't be reversed just like that.

What helps here is the approach to the ideal of the form as it is presented through the rules for posture and movement. Improvement in the performance of the movement sequence results in a "workout" of the entire body; this releases the built-up tensions and energy blockage.

The meaning of relaxation in the exercises is often underrated. Cheng Man-Ch'ing tells us that he constantly heard "Relax yourself, let go, you aren't relaxed!" from his teacher, Yang Cheng-Fu.[17] He describes the great progress he made through persistent practicing of relaxation.

He noticed that many practitioners never even consider relaxation as one of the important elements of T'ai Chi Ch'uan, and that he only knew of a few who had achieved an advanced level of relaxation.

Relaxation is closely related to the important principles of sink and root; it contributes decisively to deeper breathing and the development of Ch'i.

---

17 Chen Man-Ch'ing. *Thirteen Chapters on T'ai Chi Ch'uan,* page 100.

6. Exert No Force

In T'ai Chi Ch'uan, not the slightest force should be used . . . or do you doubt perhaps that strength can be developed in this way?

Yang Cheng-Fu

T'ai Chi Ch'uan should be practiced with as little physical effort as possible. If the movement sequences are correctly learned, the practitioners should try to perform the movements with diminishing physical effort. The attempt for more gentleness and letting go in the movement is closely connected with this.

The principle "exert no force" applies to all the exercises in T'ai Chi Ch'uan, even the partner exercises. Through the persistent attempt to fulfill this guiding principle, T'ai Chi Ch'uan differs not only from other martial arts, but also from all other exercise systems. Hsing I[18] and Pa Kua are also not directed by this principle in a comparable way.

The meaning of exert no force becomes increasingly clear for us through advanced practice: the less physical effort is used, the more clearly perceptible the flow of Ch'i becomes. Correspondingly, a conscious development and cultivation of the Ch'i can take place.

The principle exert no force shouldn't be observed in isolation any more than the other principles since it only receives its legitimacy through interplay with the other maxims.

---

18 Representative of the soft or inner school to which T'ai Chi Ch'uan and Pa Kua also belong.

7. Quotations from the Old Masters

Sun Lu-Tang (1861–1932)

"Through the development of inner energy, the human being can be led to his real nature."[19]

"T'ai Chi Ch'uan uses the existing conditions of the human body but not the physical force."[20]

"The human being finds himself in his natural state when he doesn't need to use force."[21]

Tung Ying Chieh (1888–1961)

"The gentle T'ai Chi method is the real T'ai Chi method."[22]

"We don't practice self-defense techniques to push others around but rather to train in these wonderful principles together with our friends."[23]

Chen Wei-Ming (?–1960)

"Be modest. Even when you have accomplished abilities, don't be proud. Every martial art is different. Only when you are modest can you learn about yourself and others and progress in your practicing."[24]

"The contents of T'ai Chi Ch'uan are difficult to communicate in a performance. T'ai Chi Ch'uan serves the development of the personality but not for such purposes. In order to awaken the interest of an audience, one used to rapidly demonstrate the form and the partner exercises."[25]

"When we are completely relaxed, the Ch'i can sink to the lower Tan T'ien. When we use force, this natural condition can't be attained."[26]

"If physical force is used, one can't profit from T'ai Chi Ch'uan. Even if the movements are correctly performed on the surface, one hasn't internalized the art."[27]

---

19 From an article about T'ai Chi Ch'uan by Dr. Chi published in *West and East Monthly*, 1965.
20 Ibid.
21 Ibid.
22 *Tai Chi Touchstones: Yang Family Secret Transmissions*, page 145.
23 Ibid., page 149.
24 *T'ai Chi Ch'uan Ta Wen: Questions and Answers on T'ai Chi Ch'uan*, page 47.
25 Ibid., page 46.
26 Ibid., page 41.
27 Ibid., page 42.

"When we stick to our partner and follow him unintentionally through all the changes of the movements, we experience the wonderful essence that is underlying all changes. It is the state 'without form,' in which there are no limits and no differences."[28]

Yang Cheng-Fu (1882–1936)

"The perfection of this art is not dependent on the figure and age but rather exclusively on the understanding of the practitioner. I have practiced this art for fifteen years, but all the same, I often feel the necessity of asking a teacher for advice."[29]

"Gentleness and unity of the body, mind and Ch'i are of major importance. Through your practicing, excellency will take care of itself."[30]

"Only when we understand the principles, apply them with the utmost care and internalize them completely can our art reach perfection."[31]

"When the cultivation of Ch'i comes about naturally and this process is not violated, the Ch'i will always be present. The lightness and sensitivity in humans is their spirit. When our spirit isn't pure, how can we do justice to our role as the third partner in the unity with heaven and earth? What purpose does life have when we aren't true to our real nature, to cultivate life, extend our spirit and develop ourselves positively?"[32]

---

28 Ibid., page 42.
29 *Tai Chi Touchstones: Yang Family Secret Transmissions*, page 142.
30 Ibid., page 134.
31 Ibid., page 132.
32 Ibid., pages 136–37.

8. Let Go (Release), Non-Action, and Follow

Let go, non-action, and follow are essential Taoist values. Through their practical application in T'ai Chi Ch'uan, their mental/spiritual manifestation is set upon the path. Since a literal interpretation of their meaning perhaps isn't clear enough, they shall be explained below.

Let Go (Release)

If we develop the ability to release, we can maintain quietness and composure. In everyday life, this helps us to handle the demands placed on us by our family and profession.

For our spiritual path, letting go means that the importance of mental concepts and ideas recedes into the background. From the experiences gained through practicing, we can turn our attention to what is essential.

Non-Action

The Taoist rule "action through non-action" is interpreted in various ways. It doesn't only mean that through non-action something can be influenced. It also signifies a conscious meditative action with which we do justice to things but remain free from them in spite of it.

Follow

"To withdraw and follow the other" is an important principle in the partner exercises. It requires adjusting to someone else and meeting him or her with tolerance. It also includes modesty. "Follow" doesn't mean that we give ourselves up. It has more to do with personality development as its goal by which the lower self (ego) is replaced by the higher self (true nature of humans). Also see the Tao Te Ching: "The wise man subdues his self but, all the same, he makes progress."

9. Sixty-Four Questions and Answers about T'ai Chi Ch'uan

1. Is it necessary to become acquainted with Taoist philosophy before one starts practicing?

Knowledge of Taoist philosophy is certainly helpful, but is not required for learning the exercises. The best approach to T'ai Chi Ch'uan is offered in the practice. Through this path, we arrive at an even better and more thorough understanding of Taoist teaching. It isn't limited to the intellectual approach, but becomes an intuitive understanding which naturally develops out of practicing.

2. How long does it take to learn T'ai Chi Ch'uan?

The fundamental exercises of T'ai Chi Ch'uan—the short form, the long form, and the partner exercises—can be learned in one to three years with regular instruction and practice; individual sections of the movement sequences that can be practiced alone with benefit, in a correspondingly shorter time. However, mastering the external form doesn't complete the learning process. Achieving perfection in T'ai Chi Ch'uan through continuous inclusion of the principles takes many years, if not decades.

3. How long should one practice daily?

Even twenty minutes of daily practice brings many noticeably positive physical and mental results. For perfection in T'ai Chi Ch'uan, however, practicing for several hours over a longer period, daily if possible, is necessary.

4. What does "T'ai Chi Ch'uan" mean?

T'ai Chi (the great pole, the supreme ultimate, the mother of Yin and Yang) is synonymous with the Tao. *Ch'uan* means hand or fist. The name *T'ai Chi Ch'uan* results logically through the hand or fist, in the method of the exercise, so as to be attuned with the Tao. "T'ai Chi" is the abbreviation commonly used in the West for T'ai Chi Ch'uan. In China, "T'ai Chi Ch'uan" is only known by its complete name.

5. Is the development of Ch'i dependent on age or talent?

The development and cultivation of Ch'i can be started at any age. A specific talent isn't required. However, in the beginning the practitioners for whom softness and letting go are easier will experience the Ch'i sooner.

6. It is almost impossible for beginners to practice without making mistakes. Can this possibly be harmful?

The correct performance of a larger portion of the form is usually possible only after practicing for a somewhat longer time. Therefore, practicing with errors in the beginning can't be avoided. Due to the quality of the gentle, flowing movement, however, no physical damage should be feared. A less than perfect practicing mainly limits the possible energetic impact of T'ai Chi Ch'uan, such as the development and cultivation of the Ch'i.

7. Many practitioners can only attend courses after longer intervals. What should they do when they can only remember certain parts of the form unclearly or not at all?

Practicing doesn't need to be interrupted because of this. Until the next course, the sequences can be bridged with self-made transitions. The principle of the unity of the body in movement should especially be taken into consideration while doing this.

8. How can T'ai Chi Ch'uan be included in daily life?

Through regular practice, T'ai Chi flows by itself into our daily life. The many developments and the harmony-bringing effects that result from practicing lead to a composure that naturally allows us to better handle the affairs of daily life.

9. Can moods and feelings be expressed through T'ai Chi Ch'uan?

Though T'ai Chi Ch'uan is an art of moving, it isn't expressive dance. Doing T'ai Chi isn't a way to show moods and feelings. It is better to compare it with sitting meditation, where the attention is completely focused on practicing.

10. Does practicing T'ai Chi Ch'uan have a positive effect on creativity?

The developments brought forth through practicing contribute to creative work.
    Many artists—painters, dancers, musicians, singers, and actors—speak about how T'ai Chi Ch'uan has increased their creativity.

11. Are there special exercises in T'ai Chi Ch'uan for the treatment of specific illnesses?

T'ai Chi Ch'uan—like traditional Chinese medicine—sees illness not as an isolated process, but rather as the expression of a disturbance in the functioning of the entire body. Creating an optimal situation for the complete bodily function is, therefore, the best prerequisite for recovery. The necessary positive impact on health for this result in T'ai Chi Ch'uan comes from practicing the forms (short form, long form). Exercises for specific health problems are not a part of T'ai Chi Ch'uan.

12. Are there styles that are appropriate for one person and not for another?

A quality T'ai Chi, geared toward the principles, is suitable for everyone in the same way and can be practiced with the same success. Interestingly enough, many practitioners believe, however, that exactly the directions of styles that vary from the principles are particularly appealing. For example, they are attracted to a dynamic and power-emphasizing way of moving. Others prefer interpretations of T'ai Chi Ch'uan that aren't connected to a set form, or they favor convoluted and uncoordinated movements. These kinds and similar deviations from the principles are found to be especially appealing only because they allow practitioners to retain their habitual patterns of movement.

13. When can one teach T'ai Chi Ch'uan?

A teacher should have clear knowledge of the movement sequences and, when possible, should be so advanced that he can lead his students to a conscious development and cultivation of Ch'i.

Since there is a great demand for teachers, many practitioners teach with little T'ai Chi experience. They shouldn't neglect their own further learning.

14. Why is T'ai Chi Ch'uan also called "scholar-boxing" in China?

The description "scholar-boxing" can first be explained by the extensive treasure of knowledge and experience upon which foundation T'ai Chi Ch'uan has been developed. Secondly, it refers to the methods of T'ai Chi Ch'uan. While other disciplines accomplish their goal mainly through the repetition of physical movement sequences, T'ai Chi Ch'uan reaches the higher levels only through practicing that includes mental awareness as a major element.

In addition, even with the best of instruction perfection in T'ai Chi Ch'uan can only be accomplished through an intensive mental analysis of the material learned.

15. Can the sequence of the positions be changed at one's own discretion?

The order of the positions and the connecting transitions has no hidden meaning. For example, they aren't related to the progressive or destructive cycle of the five elements—fire, water, air, earth, and metal—as in other disciplines. They mainly follow the principle of Yin and Yang: after moving forward (attack) follows a backward retreat (yield); after a lifting, a sinking, and on on.

The sequence of the positions can, therefore, be changed, assuming that the continuous application of the principle of Yin and Yang is retained. In this way, the form creations of the styles' founders have been changed, for example, eliminating the repetitions or through readjustments. However, the experience and knowledge contained in the forms of the major styles offer the guarantee that the advanced levels of T'ai Chi Ch'uan can be reached. Each change should only be undertaken when the practitioner is highly advanced himself.

16. Is a comparison of the forms even possible?

Since all the styles refer to the classical treatises, it is possible to compare the forms of one style as well as the forms of different styles. In order to compare forms that aren't established by photographs, drawings, or descriptions, one must see them performed by a qualified teacher or a very good student. It is almost impossible to judge from a form demonstrated by a beginner.

A comparison of forms only works together with a comprehensive knowledge of the principles and techniques. Without this information, only superficial comparisons are possible. The deeper meaning—why this, that, or something else is done—remains hidden.

17. What does the demonstration of the form show?

The performance of a form reveals the knowledge about T'ai Chi Ch'uan. It makes clear how far the practitioner has incorporated the principles. Also the knowledge about the techniques and the already invested practice time are clearly noticeable.

18. Is it advisable to practice several styles at the same time?

Practicing one good style is sufficient to cause all of the effects for which T'ai Chi Ch'uan is known. Experience has shown that regular practice of many different forms prevents one from achieving depth in what is learned.

19. Should one become acquainted with other styles?

To arrive at a deeper understanding of T'ai Chi Ch'uan, a comparison of the styles is very helpful.

It is recommended, however, to search for the teachers of other style directions only when the practitioner is advanced. One must have a trained eye for the meaning which is based on the principles behind the sequences of the movements. Otherwise, one will only become confused by the differences of the forms. The individual can also only learn when he or she is open. If one considers only what one himself has learned to be good and correct, one could possibly stand in the way of one's own progress.

20. Methods foreign to T'ai Chi Ch'uan are frequently incorporated into practice. Is this procedure advisable?

Experience shows that additional exercises are usually incorporated when knowledge of T'ai Chi Ch'uan is limited. For example, the lower T'an Tien can supposedly be developed more rapidly by intense contracting and releasing of the abdominal wall. In order to use self-defense sooner and more effectively, it is advised, for example, to practice pushing an object away one hundred times daily. These and other methods contradict the natural path of T'ai Chi Ch'uan. Now the question might arise why such methods shouldn't be incorporated when, by doing so, faster results could perhaps be achieved. The classical texts warn specifically about this path: practitioners should proceed step by step. Striving for the heights without first developing the fundament is described as a widespread mistake. For a limited period of time, through using those previously named and similar methods one might achieve faster and perhaps even more spectacular results. When seen in the larger scheme of things, however, they inhibit the very development that T'ai Chi Ch'uan offers. They interfere with the refinement, and instead of opening, they harden.

Additional exercises are, therefore, only suggested when they are in harmony with the natural path of T'ai Chi Ch'uan.

21. What does "T'ai Chi-Kung Fu" mean?

In China, it is an old tradition that followers of a martial art acquire knowledge about different disciplines. In this way, T'ai Chi Ch'uan's exercises are also practiced within the various different directions of the martial arts. In this milieu, however, T'ai Chi Ch'uan is usually understood as a fighting sport and is adapted to the way of moving and the use of self-defense of each system respectively. In T'ai Chi Ch'uan, these modifications are called "T'ai Chi-Kung Fu." It is especially widespread in China, Southeast Asia, Taiwan, and Hong Kong.

22. What are the differences between Chi Kung and T'ai Chi Ch'uan?

"Chi Kung" is a collective term for mostly old Chinese exercises that activate the Ch'i. It includes a great variety of exercises. Most of the Chi Kung exercises, unlike in T'ai Chi Ch'uan, are specifically applied exercises for health that can be performed while resting or in motion.

There are also meditative Chi Kung exercises, the so-called martial art Chi Kung, and acrobatic Chi Kung. Many of these exercises are oriented on human nature as in the sense of T'ai Chi Ch'uan. They lead to a deeper natural breathing and are directed in a similar way to letting go and relaxing. Others have moved far away from this direction. When we use the name Chi Kung as the generic term for exercises that lead to the development of Ch'i, then we can also regard T'ai Chi Ch'uan as a type of Chi Kung. Due to the uniqueness of T'ai Chi Ch'uan in the organization and performance of its exercises and its special orientation to the spirit of the Tao, such an association, however, would normally not be considered. T'ai Chi Ch'uan is viewed as an independent exercise system.

23. Is it important to regularly consult a teacher?

It is often assumed that with the movement sequences, everything essential in T'ai Chi Ch'uan has been learned. If T'ai Chi Ch'uan is being practiced solely for health reasons and relaxation, then this could be true. But when the practitioners want to progress further and possibly teach others themselves, they should visit a competent teacher at regular intervals. All too easily, we fall back into old movement habits in our practicing. We also tend toward performing the movements inaccurately. That is especially the case when no clarity exists about the self-defense techniques contained within the movements. Even when we sense that our practicing is beneficial for us, our progress could be affected.

In addition, we tend to overestimate our abilities. Having corrections by a teacher time and time again makes us aware of our actual level of development.

A deepening of what one learns is almost unobtainable without a qualified teacher. His corrections and instructions have decisive importance. They lead us through an increasingly refined way of practicing to a consciously guided development and cultivation of the Ch'i.

24. Is it advisable to study with various teachers?

Learning T'ai Chi Ch'uan with various teachers is a common practice. Many masters of T'ai Chi Ch'uan had several teachers. (T. T. Liang mentions twenty!) Learning from teachers of different style directions, however, sets limits through their distinctive forms. A change of teachers within the same style is, therefore, less problematic because the forms are usually more similar.

25. What characterizes the relationship between teacher and student?

Between teacher and student is usually an open and friendly relationship; dependency and exaggerated attachment are unusual. The student goes his or her own way in harmony with the Taoist tradition, free and personally responsible.

The teacher tries to encourage the student in the best possible way. (See Tung Ying Chieh: "Master Yang Cheng-Fu was equally open and generous in teaching all his students.") However, in T'ai Chi Ch'uan he is not necessarily also the spiritual teacher, as is usual in other Eastern paths. And so, for example, it's not seen as his responsibility to guide the student to spiritual experiences. The teacher only creates, by conveying the exercises, the conditions through which they can occur.

26. Regular practicing isn't easy to achieve. Is there something that can be said to motivate someone to practice?

As in all spiritual paths, in T'ai Chi Ch'uan there are also limits for an outside motivation.

Normally some time is needed before practicing occupies a regular place in daily life and is as natural as eating and drinking. Until this point is achieved, reluctance and laziness must be overcome. At times, interest in the exercises is reduced when learning the forms is complete. (Cheng Man-Ch'ing: "Many return from a mountain full of wealth with empty hands.") Usually the motivation, however, grows with increased practice; positive experience and development motivate one to progress further forward.

It is important to view practicing as something that accompanies our entire life. Difficulties in practicing regularly are not unusual. Practicing less for a time—or sometimes not at all—can even lead to important experiences about what practicing means to us and the path attached to it.

27. What considerations could help prevent competitive thoughts and judgment about the development of other practitioners?

Each individual passes through an entirely personal process of development; therefore, there is no need to observe the progress of others. It would be better to consider our practice under the aspect that we are not only doing something for our own personal development but also making a contribution to the development of humanity.

28. Are there special exercises in T'ai Chi Ch'uan to develop Ch'i?

The posture and movement principles, as well as the design of the movement sequences are geared in a quality T'ai Chi toward achieving the best possible Ch'i development. Practicing the forms and the partner exercises based on them provides the conditions for a Ch'i development in the sense of T'ai Chi Ch'uan.

29. When does a skill in T'ai Chi Ch'uan actually exist?

A skill in T'ai Chi can only be spoken about when it is developed through the methods belonging to T'ai Chi. For example, when T'ai Chi Ch'uan is begun after practicing a different discipline for decades, the abilities that have already been acquired are naturally included in T'ai Chi. Individual abilities, for example, such as pushing an opponent away for more than several meters, awaken the impression that this practitioner also possesses outstanding abilities in T'ai Chi Ch'uan. A trained observer, however, will see that a different method stands behind these results.

30. What about the claim that several months of training in the martial art Chi Kung should precede the practicing of T'ai Chi Ch'uan and that only in this manner can one come to an effective practicing of T'ai Chi?

Like in every other training system, T'ai Chi also has a specific manner of practicing and special effects connected with it. This development begins with the first step in T'ai Chi, but can naturally only be achieved through practicing in the T'ai Chi Ch'uan manner. A different type of training can, therefore, hardly have the necessary conditions for T'ai Chi practicing.

Such well-meaning recommendations and similar ones could indicate a limited knowledge of T'ai Chi Ch'uan. Through the inclusion of other training systems, there is an attempt to compensate for missing information about T'ai Chi Ch'uan in order to arrive at a more effective way of practicing.

31. There are Taoist exercises through which the small heavenly circle[33] can be opened after a few months. As a rule, when practicing T'ai Chi Ch'uan this is usually only possible after many years. Does this suggest that T'ai Chi Ch'uan is less effective than these exercises?

In T'ai Chi Ch'uan, great emphasis is placed on a natural opening of the small heavenly circle. It occurs in the Ch'i level when the development of the Ch'i and the lower Tan T'ien are very advanced. If the opening occurs in a natural fashion, it is free from the negative side effects that can easily appear from opening the circles too rapidly.[34] In addition, it has considerable meaning for spiritual development.

When the planned opening of the heavenly circles is selected as a meditation path, one must be prepared for an equally long practice as in every other exercise system with a comparable objective. In order to produce a lasting effect, the opening of the heavenly circles must be maintained and extended through continuous practice. Prerequisite for successful results in this, as in T'ai Chi Ch'uan, are the development of natural breathing, good posture, mature mental collectedness, and the ability to deeply relax.

32. Is additional sitting meditation necessary in order to obtain a higher level in T'ai Chi Ch'uan?

T'ai Chi Ch'uan and sitting meditation, such as Zazen (Zen Buddhism) or Taoist meditation, are often combined. To arrive at a higher level of T'ai Chi, however, it isn't necessary to practice additional sitting meditation.

---

33 The small heavenly circle moves along the spinal column, following the upward path of the wonder meridian *Tu Mo* and downward on the centerline of the body, following the path of the wonder meridian *Yen Mo*. It is considered open when Tu Mo and Yen Mo join in one circle and the circulation of the Ch'i is clearly discernable in them.

34 The opening of the small heavenly circle follows the opening of the so-called large heavenly circle, in which additional important meridians are opened and connected.

33. Is it sensible to practice T'ai Chi Ch'uan together with other methods, such as Hatha Yoga or Zazen?

Although all of the above-mentioned methods have different approaches and place other priorities, they all work on deep breathing, relaxation, and development in the subtle energy realm. That's why they can be practiced together. However, experience has shown that when one is more advanced, one tends to concentrate on one practice method due to time limitations. In order to perfect one of the named paths, not only is it necessary to concentrate all of one's energies on a particular practice method, but also a great deal of time is needed.

34. Is there a confirmation about the levels of development one achieves in T'ai Chi Ch'uan?

A confirmation about the levels of development through tests doesn't exist in T'ai Chi Ch'uan as it does in other disciplines, for example, as is customary in karate. In T'ai Chi one assumes that all levels of development speak for themselves, so to speak. To confirm this through tests and titles has never been considered necessary at any point in the history of T'ai Chi Ch'uan.[35]

35. What significance do the handed-down records of lineage have?

The records of lineage handed down in the T'ai Chi Ch'uan literature give us a picture of T'ai Chi from its beginnings to today's teachers. Since it isn't common in T'ai Chi Ch'uan to name a direct successor, the records of lineage only bear a selection of important teachers. They show one or more master students of a well-known teacher who have especially distinguished themselves through their abilities.

36. What is meant in T'ai Chi Ch'uan by a "direct transmission"?

The prerequisite for such a direct transmission is that the teacher not only has external knowledge about the advanced art of T'ai Chi at his disposal but also that this has been internalized by decades of practicing. On the basis of his development and experiences, the teacher can guide his student to a deep direct understanding. This usually refers to individual details of the exercises.

37. How does the dissemination of T'ai Chi Ch'uan occur?

Up until now the spread of T'ai Chi Ch'uan has occurred without a concerted effort of organization. For example, there are no associations that represent its different styles. Since there are no confirmations of the development levels, and it isn't common in the individual styles to name a successor, in the final analysis every teacher only represents his own approach to T'ai Chi Ch'uan. The old Taoist principle emphasizing individuality and freedom of the individual is very clearly shown here.

---

35 Correspondingly, there is no training to become a teacher of T'ai Chi Ch'uan. Practitioners teach in arrangement with their teachers when they have acquired a fundamental knowledge of T'ai Chi Ch'uan. But they remain students themselves for a long time.

38. How can mastery in T'ai Chi Ch'uan be identified?

Usually we speak of mastery when the practitioner has developed the abilities that are accredited to the Ch'i level (see page 53). When we hear about a T'ai Chi master, we normally assume that this person has the appropriate knowledge and ability at his or her disposal. However, we should realize that there is no appointment to master in T'ai Chi Ch'uan. Every practitioner can be called a T'ai Chi master by others or call himself a T'ai Chi master. There is no authority that determines whether this takes place correctly.

39. What connection exists between mastery in T'ai Chi Ch'uan and spiritual experiences?

When one uses the title "master" in T'ai Chi, it is usually associated with abilities in self-defense, such as the use of Ch'i, the mastery of self-defense techniques, and the correct performance of the forms.

This means that mastery exists in connection with the command of the exercises—the method. Such accomplishments are usually combined with a multitude of experiences. They refer to the perception of the Ch'i and the effects allied with it, as well as the perception of the subtle energy centers, especially the lower Tan T'ien and so on. The spiritual goal of T'ai Chi, to be in harmony with the Tao, goes, however, much further than these types of energy experiences.

40. How can the practice of gentle, slow, and flowing movement be of value in self-defense?

The gentle, slow, and flowing practice method is an essential element in T'ai Chi Ch'uan. It also serves to set certain developments on their way. In combination with the other principles, they encourage the balanced flexibility and elasticity of the body and, as a special result, responsiveness. In the applied use in self-defense, this makes an exceptional rapidity possible. The slow and flowing exercise method also contributes to a general strengthening of the body and plays a decisive role in the development and cultivation of Ch'i, whose application possibilities are considerably superior to physical force. Self-defense techniques applied in rapid movement and reacting directly to them are practiced in the partner exercises.

41. Can the practice of a "hard" self-defense discipline be a meaningful supplement to the practice of "soft" T'ai Chi Ch'uan?

For those who are interested in perfection in the meaning of T'ai Chi Ch'uan, the practice of a "hard" self-defense discipline is not to be recommended. The path of T'ai Chi is so completely bonded with letting go and the renunciation of the use of muscular power that a discipline focusing in the opposite direction would influence all the effects of T'ai Chi Ch'uan.

42. Are women at a disadvantage to men in self-defense in T'ai Chi Ch'uan?

T'ai Chi Ch'uan is one of the few martial arts in which body size and muscular power have no authoritative meaning. The deciding point is primarily the Ch'i development. Women can, therefore, achieve the same development as men in all areas of T'ai Chi Ch'uan.

43. If one is primarily interested in T'ai Chi Ch'uan's meditative aspect, how intensely must one concern oneself with its self-defense aspect?

All the positions contained in the movement sequences are based on self-defense techniques. The names of many positions indicate the technique that it contains: Press, Push, Ward-Off, and so on. In order to clearly and consciously perform the movement sequences, it is, therefore, extremely helpful to have a fundamental knowledge of the techniques contained in them. The necessary effort in this case is minimal. The techniques that are frequently concealed in the slow flowing manner of moving are easy to identify with some training.[36]

Quality T'ai Chi Ch'uan is always performed meditatively. Ignoring the self-defense aspect doesn't make T'ai Chi more meditative, but rather only leads to a lack of clarity about the movement sequences and to a considerable watering down of the exercises when performed. On the other hand, without clarity about the movement sequences, it's difficult to carry out any advanced practice. Also, a more advanced level in meditation can't be reached without it.

44. How much must one concern oneself with the self-defense techniques and meditation when one wants to practice T'ai Chi Ch'uan mainly for health reasons?

This is similar to the previous section. T'ai Chi can have a better effect on overall health when a meditative state of mind in practicing is cultivated and the exercises are clearly grasped with the help of a fundamental knowledge of the self-defense techniques.

Nevertheless, many positive health effects already show up when only some fundamental principles, such as a slow, flowing, and relaxed way of moving, are followed.

45. In the T'ai Chi Ch'uan literature, the exercises are often divided into levels: the solo exercises, partner exercises, Ta Lu, sword and pole forms. Does this mean that the short form or the long form is less important for advanced practice?

This division shouldn't be misunderstood. The solo exercises (short form and long form) always remain fundamental for practicing. The partner exercises and the Ta Lu are primarily described as advanced because practicing them makes more sense when the individual has progressed further. Practicing the pole and sword forms isn't necessary for perfection in T'ai Chi. Exercising with the sword is even seen as an independent way of practice.

We shouldn't forget that the same principles apply in all the exercises. Seen from this point of view, there are no exercises only for beginners or advanced practitioners.

46. Does the division of the styles into "Yin" and "Yang" exist in T'ai Chi Ch'uan?

This kind of approach to the styles isn't possible in T'ai Chi Ch'uan, since a style can't be entirely Yin or Yang. Such a division is only possible for individual elements or components of a style. The same elements can be Yin or Yang in the different styles. Others are always Yin or, respectively, Yang in order to be fair to the essence of T'ai Chi Ch'uan; still others must contain the balance of Yin and Yang. Following are a few examples.

---

36 Knowledge about the "outer" form of the self-defense techniques is meant here. The application of the techniques in the partner exercises, for example, is considerably more difficult.

The outer appearance of a style can be described as Yin when it is distinguished by large reaching movements, and as Yang when it is distinguished by smaller, more compact movements.

In comparison, the gentle, soft specific way of moving in T'ai Chi Ch'uan is always Yin. See Cheng Man-Ch'ing: "Through pure Yin (greatest possible softness and suppleness), the highest Yang (stability and strength) is achieved." A dynamic, sporty, strongly performed T'ai Chi can be described as Yang, although this way of moving isn't compatible with the principles of T'ai Chi Ch'uan.

The creation of the movement sequences orients itself in a quality T'ai Chi Ch'uan, on the other hand, on a balance of Yin and Yang (in alteration of the movements from forward and backward, up and down, lift and sink, and so on).

47. What importance do the forms have?

The forms are supposed to make it possible to practice according to the principles. They are helpers, tools. They aren't rigidly set movement combinations, but rather flexible within the framework of the principles.

48. How can the different adjustments of the principles in the forms be explained?

Advanced levels of T'ai Chi can only be achieved when a comprehensive knowledge accompanies a readiness to get involved with practicing in the sense of T'ai Chi Ch'uan. However, the practitioners, occasionally even the sons and daughters of the great masters, are sometimes missing the meaning of the important principles that should be included in the practice. If the principles aren't incorporated into practicing in the necessary way, no deeper, thorough understanding of the exercises can occur. When forms develop or rather modulate from this foundation, they show themselves, for instance, in a way of moving that is more about holding on rather than letting go; techniques that are only intent on effectiveness without orienting themselves on the principles of optimal body movement (health aspect), or that the movement sequences have lost their uniformity and special coordination.

49. Why is the alignment of the principles on the nature of human beings an important key to understanding the exercises?

This orientation explains, among other things, why the principles are coordinated and compatible in their effects upon each other. They make the timelessness of the forms clear. Their quality isn't dependent on age but rather on the degree of alignment with the principles.

It lets the method of T'ai Chi be known: individual abilities aren't strived for but result instead in a natural way from practicing.

50. What do the so-called secrets mean?

The "secrets" are the less well-known explanations about the principles. They refer to the shape as well as to the performance of the movement sequences. A more refined exercising and, therefore, a more effective Ch'i development is possible by following them. This valuable knowledge is still described today as secret, even if it is openly passed on, to emphasize its importance.

51. What should the proportion be for "practice in motion" and "practice in non-motion"?

T'ai Chi Ch'uan is connected to practice in motion. All the effects attributed to it occur from the developments of practice in motion and can also only be accomplished through this. Practicing in a quiet position—as in "Zen standing,"[37] for example, or in holding individual positions—can certainly be included. This strengthens the legs and helps to center the energy, as in sitting meditation. To spend more practice time on holding positions rather than in movement, however, is not in harmony with the ideas of T'ai Chi Ch'uan.

Also, poor posture can be corrected better through a continually improved performance of the form in motion than through a correction in standing. Practicing in motion especially establishes the specific comprehensive results of T'ai Chi. When the individual stands more in his practicing than he moves, the exceptional possibilities of T'ai Chi Ch'uan aren't being used.

52. Is it advisable to practice the solo forms not only to the right, but also to the left (mirror image)?

The fact that we begin the solo exercises with the weight shifted onto the right foot doesn't mean that in the following movement sequences the right side of the body is more involved than the left. This would be contrary to the ideas of T'ai Chi Ch'uan. The positions in a quality T'ai Chi are always organized so that both sides of the body are proportionally challenged and can develop independently whether the exercise was started to the right or to the left. It is, therefore, enough to practice the exercises starting to one side, which usually happens to be the right. There are teachers, however, who place great value on practicing the form to both sides.

The hypothesis that only exercise that begins to the right is beneficial for the Ch'i development is without any foundation. It is also not necessary to recommend practicing to the left for women or left-handers.

53. Does T'ai Chi Ch'uan develop body consciousness?

A perfection in the T'ai Chi sense isn't imaginable without a developed body awareness. The principles are, therefore, also aimed at developing it. Through the Ch'i development, a dimension of body awareness arises that is beyond what is normally understood under body awareness. Body consciousness arises in T'ai Chi Ch'uan not only out of the awarely experienced movement of the body. It emerges, on the contrary, when the posture and movement can be distinctly felt and carried from the inner energy. This leads to the development of a deep and lasting body awareness that is a prerequisite for a comprehensive consciousness and attentiveness.

---

[37] Zen standing: You stand in the parallel stance, both arms in a rounded position at chest level.

54. How long did the old masters practice?

There are few exact accounts about how long the old masters practiced daily. It is said that the masters of the Chen-style, for example, practiced the long form at least twenty times daily—which can take about four hours. It is known that for Yang Cheng-Fu, twelve times the long form comprised the foundation of his daily practice. As he said himself, there were also times when he practiced day and night.

What is certain is that the higher levels of development require decades of regular practice. At the same time, as for all practitioners, next to periods of intensive practicing there were also ones where considerably less was practiced.

55. Can one perceive Ch'i?

During advanced practice, the movement of the Ch'i becomes constantly clearer: One feels the movement of the Ch'i in the weight shifts; one can guide the Ch'i mentally; the sinking and rising of the Ch'i is experienced. The general accumulation of the Ch'i is strongly felt in the body as well as the circulation of the Ch'i in the meridians, as it occurs in the opening of the heavenly circles.

56. How can T'ai Chi Ch'uan be understood as a breathing exercise?

A conscious coordination of breathing with movement only makes sense when the practitioner is more advanced. Without including deep breathing, which is also known as a main carrier of Ch'i, it isn't possible to attain a higher Ch'i development in T'ai Chi Ch'uan. All the principles are, therefore, directed to provide the best possible conditions for breathing. The increased softness and flexibility deepens breathing in a natural way. The abdominal breathing that ensues in this way creates the optimal conditions for the so-called "Ch'i breathing" by which the cosmic energy is breathed in and out, so to speak, accompanying the breathing process of the lungs.

57. What effect does T'ai Chi Ch'uan have on the system of meridians?

Practicing causes:

1. An activation of the flow of energy in the entire system of meridians.[38]

2. A special stimulation of the stream of energy in *those* meridians that correspond in their direction with the wide-flowing Ch'i (see page 51).[39]

3. An intensifying of the stream of energy in various meridians through the special structure of the positions. For example, the opening of the wonder meridian Tu Mo is supported through the practice of the position "Step Back and Repulse Monkey."

---

38 T'ai Chi Ch'uan includes the results of many known Eastern exercise systems that cause an activation of the Ch'i through massage or various body and breathing exercises.

39 The twelve main meridians are divided into six yin and six yang meridians. The yin meridians move from bottom to top; the yang meridians from top to bottom.

During practice, however, one doesn't concentrate on the individual meridians in order to activate the stream of energy in them, as is known in Chi Kung and in the Taoist meridian meditation. In the use of Ch'i in self-defense, energy is also not directed through the meridians.

For a better understanding, we must clearly differentiate between the energy course in the meridians and the movement of Ch'i caused by practicing T'ai Chi Ch'uan.

The meridian system, which holds a key position in physical and mental health, works continually. The stream of energy in the meridians flows in a specific direction and is limited to the paths of energy.

On the other hand, the movement of the Ch'i caused by practicing T'ai Chi Ch'uan begins and ends with practicing. It is perceived as wide flowing. It is part of the phenomenon that is called "the big cosmic Ch'i." It is this Ch'i that in its pure unconditional form permeates animate and inanimate nature and maintains all life.

Experience confirms here that it has to do with various phenomena: while practicing the form, the perceived opening of a meridian is experienced independently from the movement and direction of the broad-flowing Ch'i.[40]

58. What changes have been caused by the rapid spread of T'ai Chi Ch'uan?

The exceedingly rapid spread of T'ai Chi Ch'uan during the past century (millions of practitioners in China alone) has led to an extensive watering down of the exercises. Next to the old styles that are still practiced, there are an almost incalculable variety of exercises derived from them. These exercises are also called T'ai Chi Ch'uan but can't be assigned to any style. They are generally based only on a few fundamental principles. Frequently, they are mixed with different exercise systems. Even the practice of individual movement sequences is often considered to be full-value T'ai Chi Ch'uan. (This development in China has gone so far that every exercise that is performed slowly and relaxed and can't be classified is called T'ai Chi.) The watering down of the exercises can't only be traced back to the fact that the real T'ai Chi was kept secret by some of the initiated. It can more easily be explained from the complexity of the T'ai Chi method. A thorough understanding is only possible after extensive practice over a longer period of time. Therefore, the rapid spread of T'ai Chi Ch'uan occurred without enough time to prepare qualified teachers.

59. Does an exercise like T'ai Chi, which favors gradual change, have little to offer to Western students who expect fast results?

The implication that T'ai Chi attaches importance to gradual changes can be explained by the realization that habits that have hardened over decades can only be successfully and lastingly reversed over a longer period of time.[41] Also the correction of poor posture and the movement habits arising from it, in connection with the spiritual and emotional processes of change, can be worked through better by the individual if this doesn't

---

40 A meridian is considered "open" when the stream of energy in it can be clearly perceived.
41 See also *Speeches and Parables of Tschuang-Tse*, page 14: "You go too fast. You get an egg and you already want to hear it crow. You pull your crossbow and you already want to have a roast duck in front of you."

happen too rapidly but rather gradually.[42] This doesn't mean that there aren't any rapid results in T'ai Chi. Many practitioners report about remarkable changes after only a short time. The pleasant harmonizing effects of the exercises in general are noticeable from the beginning.

60. Why is it often difficult to understand the exercises?

A main reason for this lies in the many aspects of T'ai Chi. The fact that many practitioners today are only interested in one aspect of T'ai Chi Ch'uan and many teachers only have the ability to pass on one aspect of T'ai Chi has resulted in a primarily one-sided knowledge about T'ai Chi.

For the followers of T'ai Chi-Kung Fu, T'ai Chi is purely a martial art. For the practitioners who understand T'ai Chi as a martial art, the meditative exercise has almost no meaning. It has only a subordinate role, if any at all. Practitioners who only see T'ai Chi as a health exercise have problems understanding T'ai Chi Ch'uan as meditation and self-defense. The representatives of a meditative T'ai Chi, on the other hand, often consider self-defense as a rather foreign aspect and would like to be completely freed of it. For all of these practitioners, the many connections concerning the exercises stay without explanation and a comprehensive understanding of T'ai Chi Ch'uan can't be reached.

61. How should we consider the claim that the goal of T'ai Chi Ch'uan, harmony with the Tao, can also be accomplished without practicing the forms but in a purely mental way and exactly such an approach is the real path upon which T'ai Chi Ch'uan was founded?

The path of T'ai Chi Ch'uan is always connected with practicing its forms in agreement with the principles. Only through practicing the forms can the special development be guided on the way that in T'ai Chi Ch'uan's own manner leads to harmony with the Tao. By an approach to the same goal in a purely intellectual way, it would be incorrect to speak of T'ai Chi Ch'uan.

62. Should one try to influence someone who is obviously practicing a watered-down T'ai Chi Ch'uan?

Since the individual usually strongly identifies with what he practices, having an influence is extremely problematic. Only when someone expresses doubt himself or questions, should one try to advise him.

63. What should be especially taken to heart by the practitioner?

The willingness to continue learning and to time and again check one's own performance of the exercises is of greatest importance for advancement in T'ai Chi.

64. Why does perfection in T'ai Chi Ch'uan often appear to be unattainable for beginners?

In the first years of practicing, our progress often appears to be slow. When, as it says in the classical texts, "the foundation has been laid," that means that the principles have been internalized to a certain extent, breathing has deepened in a natural way and the Ch'i is perceived in movement, progress receives a new dynamic and goes noticeably faster."

---

42 In modern Western body therapy, one speaks in this case about "muscle armor." In its individual effect, for example, it's possible to "read" in an extreme tightness in the shoulders and neck the basic problems of each person.

10. Meditation

Meditative practice in T'ai Chi refers, in general, to the following two methods:

- Practice with complete attention[43]
- Concentration on the lower Tan T'ien[44]

The first method is used in practicing the forms, Push Hands, and the application of the techniques. In this way, the unity of the movement of the body, breath, and Ch'i and the performance of the individual principles are carried out with full attention.

The second method, which is one of the most important Taoist meditation practices, is suggested by various teachers especially for the performance of the forms. Cheng Man-Ch'ing, for example, placed great value on practicing the short form with attention on the lower Tan T'ien.[45]

Both methods can only be put into practice when the movement sequences have been clearly learned and the principles largely internalized. Then the meditative practice in the manner described here takes on an ever-increasing role. Experience shows that beginners are overtaxed by this kind of practice.

We know from the meditative practices in Hinduism, Buddhism, and Taoism that an important aspect of meditation is the development of the subtle energy Ch'i. Through this, the subtle energy realm is effected, and the spiritual development of humans is set upon the path.

That means these meditative ways represent not only particular forms of spiritual practice but are also methods of energy development. Because the subtle energy realm is the same in all human beings and the subtle energy processes follow the same inherent laws, fundamental counterparts are found in the building blocks of the traditional Eastern meditation exercises. They all work with *posture, breathing, relaxation, and mental exercise,* such as attentiveness, collectedness, contemplation, or concentration.[46] The subtle energy realm is influenced through these elements. The development (awakening) of the subtle energy centers prepares, for example, the way for spiritual experiences.

---

43 Comparable to the Shikantaza in Zen Buddhism.
44 An important subtle energy center below the navel.
45 Cheng Man-Ch'ing recommends retaining the concentration on the lower Tan T'ien in daily life, too. In this way, an essential part of the exercise is always maintained and the effect of the exercises generally intensified. See Cheng Man-Ch'ing, *Advanced T'ai Chi Form Instructions*, page 33.
46 The teachings of Tibetan Yoga, Lama Kong Ka: "There are three essentials in the Mahamudra practice: equilibrium, relaxation, and naturalness. 'Equilibrium' means to balance the body, mouth and mind. The Mahamudra way of balancing the body is to loosen it, of balancing the mouth is to slow down the breathing, and of balancing the mind is not to cling to and rely on anything. This is the supreme way to tame the body, breath (prana) and mind.

'Relaxation' means to loosen the mind, to let everything go, to strip off all the ideas and thoughts. When one's whole body and mind become loose, one can, without effort, remain in the natural state, which is intrinsically non-discriminative and yet without distractions.

'Naturalness' means not 'taking' or 'leaving' anything; in other words the yogi does not make the slightest effort of any kind. He lets the senses and mind stop or flow by themselves without assisting or restricting them. To practice naturalness is to make no effort and be spontaneous." (From *The Middle Way: Journal of the Buddhist Society*, London, Vol. 54, No. 2, 1979, page 81.)

T'ai Chi contains all the named building blocks practiced in the sitting meditation. For instance, the upright relaxed position of the torso taken in all T'ai Chi exercises corresponds to the position practiced in sitting meditation.[47] Since the torso is steadily moved as a unit forward and backward as well as turned, the best conditions are provided for deep breathing and all the subtle energy processes referring to the torso area.

Through the influence on the subtle energy realm, as it is said in T'ai Chi Ch'uan, the true nature of humans is made accessible, that is, opened.

The fact that human traits such as goodness, tolerance, wisdom, intuition, love, and awareness are developed through abstract meditation without direct effort upon them shows clearly that the spiritual nature is naturally embedded in us. In this way, the old Taoists saw the characteristics of human nature as spiritual and good.

That the spirituality is natural is also confirmed by the experiences won through practicing. The further we progress in the realization of the principles, the easier it is for us to maintain our attention while practicing. If the development of the lower Tan T'ien is well advanced, the concentration can be held there, as if by itself. The natural meditative state of mind that occurs is the fundament for comprehensive consciousness and attention. The well-known question from Zen Buddhism, "Is the Master at home?" can now be answered positively.

At this point it should be emphasized again that the "methods" of classical T'ai Chi Ch'uan are concerned with working on the principles. The best conditions for a Ch'i development, that has an extensive effect on the subtle energy realm, are seen in putting them into practice. The Ch'i development through movement (see the following) has the decisive meaning in this context.[48] The realization of the principles leads to higher levels of Taoist meditation such as the development of the golden elixir (also known as the elixir of immortality). It affects the opening of the small and large heavenly circles, the development of the subtle energy centers, and the rising of the Yang-Ch'i.[49]

The spiritual goal of T'ai Chi, however, goes even further. Through the opening and connecting of the three Tan T'iens (lower, middle, and upper), the practitioner can proceed to the experience of the "eternal spring," an ancient synonym for the Tao. The spiritual realization connected with this then leads to the oneness or harmony with the Tao. See the classical treatise *The Song of the Thirteen Postures* by Wang Tsung Yueh: "Search to know the aim of the art, the 'eternal spring' is what you may find."

---

47 See *Der Weg des T'ai Chi Ch'uan,* pages 31–38, currently only available in German.

48 An exercise primarily focused on breathing is as little in balance with the principles as a practice that deals exclusively with the opening of the meridians.

49 The rising, or shooting up, of the Yang-Ch'i (hot Ch'i) in the area of the spinal column is a phenomenon attributed to the energy movement in the large heavenly circle. The Yang-Ch'i is synonymous with the Kundalini in the Indian tradition. The rising of the Yang-Ch'i usually occurs only after the opening of the small heavenly circle that flows under the epidermis. For the Taoists, the shooting up of the Yang-Ch'i is a sign that the Ch'i development, the opening of the meridians, and the development of the three Tan T'iens are quite advanced. Essentially, this is promoted through the upright erect posture of the spinal column, as is the opening of the wonder meridian Tu Mo.

11. Energy

The Ch'i Development

The comprehensive holistic effect of T'ai Chi Ch'uan occurs in many ways out of the development of Ch'i (here meaning cosmic or inner energy)[50] and the influences associated with it in the subtle energy realm. This realm is considered to be the connecting element between the physical and the psychic/mental aspects of human beings.

Breathing, concentration, attentiveness, posture, relaxation, and movement are seen as determining factors in the Ch'i development.

Breathing

The deepening of respiration to abdominal breathing or "natural breathing" achieved through practice creates the best possible conditions for the so-called "Ch'i breathing." In it, cosmic Ch'i is "breathed" along with air during the normal breathing process. Ch'i breathing brings about the accumulation of Ch'i in the lower Tan T'ien, which stimulates and strengthens the entire subtle energy realm, including the other subtle energy centers and the flow of energy in the meridian system. It contributes considerably to the awakening of the subtle energy centers and to the natural opening of the heavenly circles.

Concentration

Concentration on the lower Tan T'ien, as practiced in T'ai Chi, effects the accumulation of Ch'i in this center and has an effect comparable to that of Ch'i breathing.

Attention

The attentive practice leads to collectedness by which the Ch'i is retained in the subtle energy realm.

The aware performance of the individual principles strengthens the Ch'i development that goes together with them.

Posture

The upright, erect posture supports the centering of the energy in the lower Tan T'ien as in the entire torso and has effects similar to Ch'i breathing.[51]

In addition, it helps to "channel" the awakened energy, for instance, in the opening of the heavenly circles and the rising of the Yang-Ch'i.

Movement

The Ch'i development through movement results mainly from the "rhythm" of the movement (Yin/Yang principle). Together with the weight shift, the energy flow becomes

---

[50] The term *Ch'i* has various meanings in Chinese. Ch'i is not only understood to be the "cosmic or inner energy," but also, among others, "breath" and "air" as well as the ability of a person to function.
[51] The developed lower Tan T'ien is similar to *Hara* in Japanese.

polarized in a special way and so strengthened. The Ch'i development through movement intensifies the subtle energy processes to a high degree. It is also the prerequisite for the use of the Ch'i in self-defense in the sense of T'ai Chi.

This method of Ch'i development points out a particular background of knowledge and experience unique to T'ai Chi Ch'uan. Even in the Taoist exercises, there is no other method that proceeds in a comparable way.

The movement of the Ch'i that accompanies the movement of the body is broadly experienced. It is felt in all the limbs of the body and the relevant half of the torso or crosses the torso in a wide path (see Advanced Practice, page 60). The movement of energy described here doesn't limit itself to the lines of energy (meridians) that are known in acupuncture or acupressure, as is often supposed. It proceeds on a less differentiating level (see questions and answers, number 57).

Ch'i and Chin

It is understood that the special abilities accompanying a developed Ch'i in T'ai Chi Ch'uan are known as individual energies (*Chin*). The training of these energies results from the practice of the movement sequences in T'ai Chi. Their application and the exact differentiation is practiced in Push Hands and Ta Lu. The various Chin can be divided into two main groups:

1. The energies that are fundamental for a refined application in T'ai Chi are: the sticking energy (*Nien Chin*), the hearing energy (*T'ing Chin*), and the yielding energy (*Tsou Chin*).

2. The energies that are connected with a performance of specific techniques, such as the uprooting or lifting energy (*T'i Chin*), the turning energy (*Chen Ssu-Chen*), and the exploding energy (*Fa Chin*).[52] The last two are characteristic for the Chen-style. In its forms, turning movements of the arms and legs are particularly emphasized. The use of the exploding energy in the Chen-style is undertaken with a sudden movement and sometimes a loud shout. This requires an advanced Ch'i development and a great softness and relaxation, otherwise the internal organs can be damaged.

---

52 See Chen Wei-Ming, *T'ai Chi Ch'uan-Ta Wen*, pages 37–39.

一

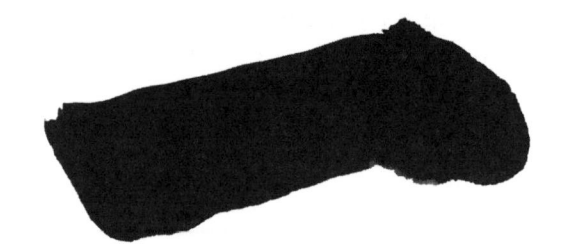

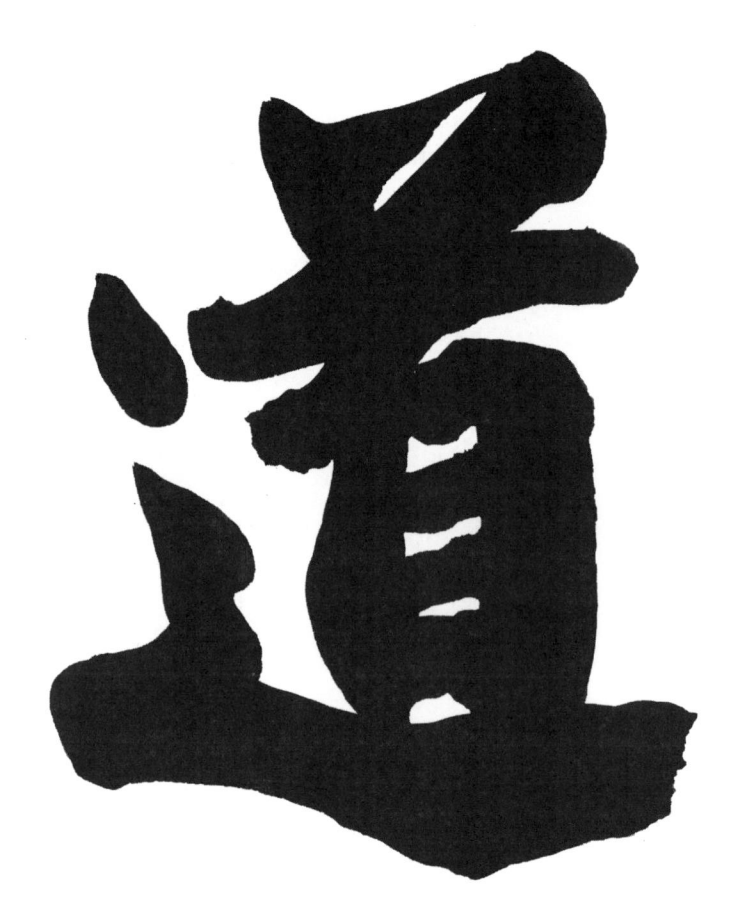

道

One way

12. Six Levels of Development

The levels of development are not uniformly set. This division into six levels helps to illustrate the process of development in T'ai Chi.[53] How long a practitioner takes to reach each level depends on the intensity of his or her practice. In order to reach the third level, the "energy level," many years of regular practice are necessary.

The individual levels are:

1. The form level or force level

Even though we try to move softly and lightly, our performance in the beginning is determined in many ways by physical strength. Only after continuous practice are the movements progressively filled and carried by Ch'i. That means that the practicing is largely limited in the beginning to the performance of the external form.

2. The technique level

This level is closely related to the first one. Practitioners at this level have completed learning the standard exercises. Since their energy development isn't advanced, the self-defense techniques cannot yet be applied using the Ch'i.

3. The energy level

At this level, the Ch'i is so far developed that it is clearly experienced during the movement. The method of practicing is continually refined. In the self-defense techniques, the Ch'i can gradually be used more often. Characteristic for the energy level is an employment of the Ch'i that is still connected with the external performance of the techniques, that is, with the movement of the body.

4. The Ch'i level

At this level, the Ch'i development is quite advanced. The Ch'i is always available and can be used independently from the techniques. The practitioner's flexibility, ability to react, and intuitive perception are extensively developed. On the Ch'i level are other important developments, too, such as the natural opening of the heavenly circles and spiritual experiences.

5. The spiritual level

"When the stage is reached in which the mind can freely move the body, then the body is liable to serve and obeys the will." This sentence from Wu Yu-Hsiang identifies the spiritual level. The body and Ch'i respond immediately in this level to the mental impulse. In order to measure how special this level is, it helps to visualize our possibilities in the beginning period. Even when we have an image of how to react to an attack, for instance, we are missing all the requirements for a reaction that identifies this level.

---

[53] Dr. Chi referred to this division. Cheng Man-Ch'ing speaks of three levels of development in his *Thirteen Chapters on T'ai Chi Ch'uan*: earth, humans, and heaven, each of which is divided again into three levels.

6. *The natural level*

At this level, as one says in T'ai Chi Ch'uan, complete physical and spiritual naturalness is achieved. Referring to the practical application of T'ai Chi, this means that on arrival in the natural level a reaction needn't be preceded by a conventional sensory perception. The practitioner reacts completely naturally. The Ch'i has grown to such an extent that it repels by itself every force directed against him.

It is important for an advancement in T'ai Chi Ch'uan sense that all the principles be included in practicing right from the beginning. For example, if letting go receives little attention, or even if force is consciously applied, then not only are the possibilities of the effect of T'ai Chi decisively interfered with but many developments occur in a manner foreign to T'ai Chi Ch'uan. A refined awareness can't take place to the same extent. Therefore, it isn't possible to come to a clear differentiation of the allied "energies" in the techniques. As a result, many areas of T'ai Chi's application remain inaccessible. A perfection in the T'ai Chi sense can't be reached. The Ch'i can only be applied in connection with physical strength. The spiritual development of the practitioner remains limited.

13. The Thirteen Basic Positions and the Techniques

At the heart of T'ai Chi Ch'uan are the so-called thirteen basic positions. These are:

> Ward-Off; Rollback; Press; Push; Split[54];
> Elbow Strike; Shoulder Push; Move Forward;
> Move Backward; Look to the Left;
> Gaze to the Right; Center Equilibrium; Pull

Ward-Off, Rollback, Press, Push, and Shoulder Push are self-defense techniques contained as positions within the forms. Ward-Off and Push are elements used in many other positions as well.[55] Split is used in the position "Lift Hands." Pull and Elbow Strike are important techniques found in the transitions connecting the positions in the forms as well as in Ta Lu.

Move Forward, Move Backward, Look to the Left, and Gaze to the Right are fundamental elements in the forms. The first two refer mainly to the weight shift. "Look to the left and gaze to the right" characterizes a perfect yielding. Only when our partner finds himself completely left or completely right of us, due to our correct yielding, can we "look to the left" or "gaze to the right."

Center Equilibrium (see page 61) is of central importance in the performance of all the positions.

The thirteen basic positions have been known since the beginning of T'ai Chi Ch'uan as its foundation. Through them, T'ai Chi in its main features is a clearly outlined exercise system. The basic positions determine the structure of the forms and, referring to the application in self-defense, the organization of practicing. The self-defense techniques contained in them are subject to the principles, as are the forms. Their external composition is geared toward an optimal body movement (health aspect), and practicing them contributes to energy development. Their application can't be separated from the correct performance of the principles.

Cheng Man-Ch'ing says, for instance, that the *true* technique should be found. By this he means that the practitioner should arrive at a correct application and clear differentiation of the individual techniques while observing the principles.

The application of the techniques always takes place in a specific connection, regardless of whether it is in Push Hands, Ta Lu, or individually practiced. In this way for instance, attacking should only follow a previous yielding.

---
54 Occasionally, "Split" is replaced by the technique "Bend Backward."
55 Push: "Single Whip," "Brush Knee," "Step Back and Repulse Monkey." Ward-Off: transition to "Single Whip," "Wave Hands in Clouds," and so on.

That means a perfect yielding is seen as the best starting position for an attack—"yielding means attacking." In this way, the important principle is kept that states "no force against force" should be used.

The techniques are an important key to understanding the exercise. When we compare the forms of teachers in a direct line of transmission, we can learn a great deal about T'ai Chi methods. Knowledge about how the same techniques are applied in various movement connections helps us to better understand the principles and to overcome the fixation that only one way is correct.

A prerequisite for the application of the techniques in the T'ai Chi Ch'uan sense is a highly developed Ch'i leading to the development of "tenacious energy" and making a distinct application of the various Chin (see page 74) possible. This also includes the knowledge of how energy can be guided, deflected, neutralized, or, for example, set free in uprooting. The muscles and sinews must first have reached the necessary flexibility so that the energy can be accumulated and then released in the same way that a bowstring is drawn. None of these developments can be forced; they need to grow through long-standing practice.

At the advanced levels, the practitioners are no longer dependent on the application of the techniques. All of their reactions have become completely natural, as one says. The principles are so internalized that they no longer require an external form in the application. The lower levels of development, however, can't be jumped over; they are an important step on the path to perfection in T'ai Chi Ch'uan.

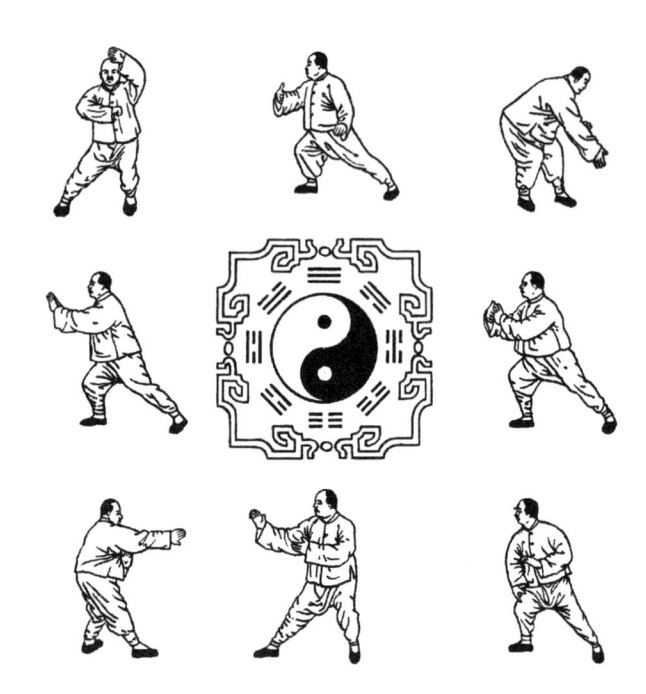

Eight Basic Positions
Elbow Strike, Ward-Off, Pull, Push, Press, Split (Bend Backward), Rollback, Shoulder Push (l-r, starting at the top left)

14. The Song of the Thirteen Positions from Yang Cheng-Fu[56]

The thirteen basic positions should always be performed with deliberation. Their center is the hips.

Undertake the change from full to empty and in reverse with great care, without losing balance. The Ch'i can then flow freely through your body without any obstacles.

If you are confronted with forceful action, meet it calmly. You can then anticipate your opponent and counter his intention.

Each individual movement should be performed with the greatest attention. In this way, the perfection will soon occur. When the lower body is completely relaxed, the Ch'i can be immediately directed outward.

If the spinal column is held upright, the "spirit of vitality" can rise to the crown of the head.

If the head is suspended from above, as if held by a string attached to the top of the head, the entire body is light and nimble in movement.

If you perform the postures carefully, bend and stretch, open and close happen as if by themselves.

Through the instruction of a qualified teacher and continual practice, excellence will come by itself.

What function does the body have in the correct performance? The answer is: the mind commands and the body obeys. Remember, the main goal of practicing is the rejuvenation and the prolongation of life.

This song of 140 characters contains all the important secrets. If you don't take them to heart, you will unfortunately lose much valuable time.

---

[56] Based on an English translation by Dr. Chi Chiang Tao.

太極拳十三勢歌訣

黎明風敬書

十三總勢莫輕視
命意源頭在腰際
變轉虛實須留意
氣遍身軀不少滯
靜中觸動動猶靜
因敵變化示神奇
勢勢存心揆用意
得來全不費工夫
刻刻留心在腰間
腹內鬆淨氣騰然

Calligraphy of the *Song of the Thirteen Positions* from Yang Cheng-Fu.

若不向此細推求,枉費工夫貽歎息。
歌兮歌兮廿四句,字字真切意無遺。
詳推用意終何在,益壽延年不老春。
若問體用何為準,意氣君來骨肉臣。
入門引路須口授,功夫無息法自修。
仔細留心向推求,屈伸開合聽自由。
尾閭中正神貫頂,滿身輕利頂頭懸。

15. Advanced Practice

When the movement sequences have been learned correctly, the principles should be intensely worked on. It is advisable when practicing to frequently direct the attention to one principle, such as, to the position of the spinal column, the position of the head, the weight shift or relaxing in the pelvic-abdominal area.

The extent to which one methodically continues remains a decision for each individual. Under no circumstance should one overexert oneself and lose the joy of practicing.

Since there are different starting levels for each individual, special attention must be devoted to specific principles. Checking oneself is as important as the regular correction by a qualified teacher. For a long time, the effort to steadily perform the principles better is an essential aspect of practicing. The ultimately strived for simultaneous application of the principles leads to the unity of body, mind, breath, and Ch'i in movement that characterizes a refined performance of T'ai Chi Ch'uan. Through continuous practice, the developments that have already taken place become accessible: the sinking of the energy is now perceptible in the movement at the end of the weight shift; the mental directing of the Ch'i is now experienced; and the subtle energy centers are noticeable as "fields of energy." Increasingly, the positive harmonizing effect of exercising is more strongly felt.

When practitioners are this advanced, they can consciously turn their attention to the development and cultivation of the Ch'i and arrive in the dimension of the higher T'ai Chi Ch'uan. Thereby the meaning of the concept of Ch'i development will also make itself accessible in a new way. The Ch'i development that one experiences can't only be attributed to one's own striving. More precisely stated, through one's own efforts, only somewhat more of the already existing immensely powerful Ch'i becomes available.

There are some principles of special importance for the Ch'i development that we shall describe below. They are the basic principles "sink," "straighten from within," "center equilibrium," and "full and empty," as well as "open and close." Only their correct application leads to the polarization of the movement without which an advanced Ch'i development can't be achieved. Through the aware performance of these basic principles, the Ch'i development will increase substantially.

Sink

The sinking of the Ch'i is a law inherent in nature. Its counterpart is the rising of the Ch'i. In Taoist teachings, these are described as the Heaven Ch'i and the Earth Ch'i. There is an ancient saying about them: "when Heaven Ch'i and Earth Ch'i are in balance, man himself is in harmony."

In a quality T'ai Chi Ch'uan, the composition and performance of the movement sequences are provided to create the best possible conditions for sinking the Ch'i. Sinking the Ch'i is connected in many ways with relaxing and letting go in the correct posture.[57] This relationship is clearly experienced in advanced practice: the more we let go, the more we perceive the sinking of the Ch'i.

Sinking the Ch'i has various results. The practitioner feels the soles of his feet stick to the ground—he is "rooted." It is an important prerequisite for the accumulation of Ch'i. For example, this is experienced at the end of the weight shift in the area of the feet like a basin filling up. The accumulation of Ch'i is also clearly perceived in the area of the lower Tan T'ien in the performance of the yielding movements.[58]

Working to sink the Ch'i, however, has to be in harmony with the rising of the Ch'i. It shall not interfere with the straightening from within that among other things, makes posture and movement easy and effortless.

Center Equilibrium ("Centered Balance")

At the beginning and the end of a weight shift, especially before all changes in direction and before setting the energy free, special attention should be paid to the center equilibrium. In its application, the sinking energy is centered (bundled) under the foot.

The center equilibrium mainly results from:

1. A slightly emphasized release in the groin area of the weight-carrying leg (see page 85).

2. It is increased through the application of the certain accents in the movement that accompany the sinking of the arms (for example, "standing hand" and relaxing the elbows).

If both are connected and performed with the necessary evenness and fineness, the practitioner clearly senses the centering of the Ch'i resulting from it.

The importance of center equilibrium can be measured by the fact that it is one of the thirteen basic positions. It extends the possibilities in self-defense to a high degree. It strengthens the "rooting" and stabilizes the balance. The concentration of energy under the foot leads, like a coiled spring, to the following mobilization of energy. Through the polarization of the movement, the center equilibrium promotes the Ch'i development.

The slight sinking at the end of the weight shift is, in the following movement, balanced again, that is, in the beginning of the shift backward through an equally small rising upward. Externally, these movements are hardly visible. In addition, they guide the practitioner, during the course of the weight shift, to depict a slightly flat curve upward and down again. The performance of center equilibrium not only spares the knee but also serves to direct the movement of the Ch'i in its course through the legs.

---

57 Cheng Man-Ch'ing describes the sinking of Ch'i as a process closely related to the relaxation of the tendons.
58 Cheng Man-Ch'ing frequently refers to the importance of the accumulation of Ch'i in the lower Tan T'ien.

Full and Empty

The shape of the form is determined in many respects by the principle of Yin and Yang.[59] This is shown by the continual weight shifts, the alternating lifting and sinking of the limbs, or by the counter-rotation of many movements. Accompanying the uniform and directed movement, this construction of the forms results in the flow of energy through the body. In each of the energy movements passing through the body, a continuous exchange of full (Yang) to empty (Yin) takes place. Therefore, there is a constant alternating aspect of Yin and Yang for each part of the body. But you might remember that the concept of "full and empty," in connection with the Ch'i movement through the body, only stands for a "more or less" of various degrees. Experience shows us that no part of the body is ever really empty, since Ch'i permeates all phenomenon of substantial and insubstantial nature.

It is easy to describe the movement of energy in the legs, since it occurs with the weight shift—the weighted leg becomes the "full" leg. The movement of energy in the arms can only be understood with knowledge about self-defense technique—the active arm performing the attack becomes the full arm, and so on.

Corresponding to the relevant technique, at the end of the weight shift the left arm and the left leg or the left leg and the right arm can be full or the other way around. In the Bow Step (see page 95), in the weight shift position moving forward, the movement of the energy proceeds as follows:[60]

>*The direct energy course:*
>The energy stays in either the right or the left side of the body. It moves, for example, from the full back foot, through the leg and the respective side of the torso, into the arm.
>Examples: Brush Right Knee, Brush Left Knee, Punch

>*The crossing energy course:*
>The energy changes from the right to the left side of the body and the reverse. It goes from the full right back foot, through the leg, crosses the torso, and then moves into the left arm.[61]
>Examples: Ward-Off, Left; Ward-Off, Right; Single Whip

Quality T'ai Chi Ch'uan shows itself in the possibility of an immediate change from full to empty. When energy is used, the full part of the body from which the energy has been set free should immediately become empty so that the opponent doesn't have the opportunity to present a counterattack. In practicing the forms, after the weight shift the

---

59 According to Taoist philosophy, from the One-Ultimate way (Tao) grows the duality (Yin and Yang). All the opposing phenomenon that make up this world can be divided into Yin and Yang.
60 We shall limit ourselves here to this description of the energy movement. The change from full and empty can also be shown in the other positions and in the connecting transitions. Such a detailed description here would be going too far.
61 Cheng Man-Ch'ing describes in his book, *Thirteen Chapters on T'ai Chi Ch'uan,* page 86, only the crossing energy course.

full arm starts to become empty again and performs the yielding that usually follows; the full arm is active, the empty arm is ready to immediately become active.

The movement of energy through the body occurs by itself in practicing a refined T'ai Chi Ch'uan. In T'ai Chi directions that only orient themselves roughly on the principles, the energy movement usually takes place solely in the legs. An application of energy for self-defense in the sense of T'ai Chi is almost impossible here because of the limited development.

Open and Close

When the Ch'i in the movement is clearly perceived, "open and close" should be practiced accompanying the weight shift. Opening usually comes into use while shifting forward (attack), and closing while shifting backward (withdraw). When closing, the energy is accumulated, compressed, concentrated; when opening, this accumulated energy is brought outward. Knowledge about the self-defense techniques contained in the positions and transitions is required for the application of opening and closing. The energy is directed to the opponent through the part of the body that comes into contact with the opponent in self-defense, that is, depending on the position, the hand, lower arm, elbows, shoulder, or foot. In the shifting backward movement that always follows, the accumulation of Ch'i occurs accompanied by breathing (opening, exhalation; closing, inhalation).

An opening, performed in this way while shifting forward, is of great importance for self-defense, since the practitioner acquires in this manner the ability to apply Ch'i over a distance, too. After every opening follows a closing which trains the accumulation of Ch'i in the area of the lower Tan T'ien and strengthens and develops, at the same time, this important subtle energy center.

It is interesting that "open and close" can also be practiced in the opposite direction of the way just described. That means in the weight shift forward, toward the end of the position, one practices compressing the energy in the parts of the body that should be used. The practitioner has the sensation of pressing against a resistance in the air! In a case of direct self-defense, this compacted potential energy would be used against the opponent. Practicing the opening while shifting backward accents the yielding element of the form, and the opponent is unable to find a point to attack. The last variation allows an effective self-defense in the first levels (see page 53), but the practitioner is not placed in the position to use Ch'i over a distance that characterizes an advanced level of T'ai Chi Ch'uan.

平 均
正 匀

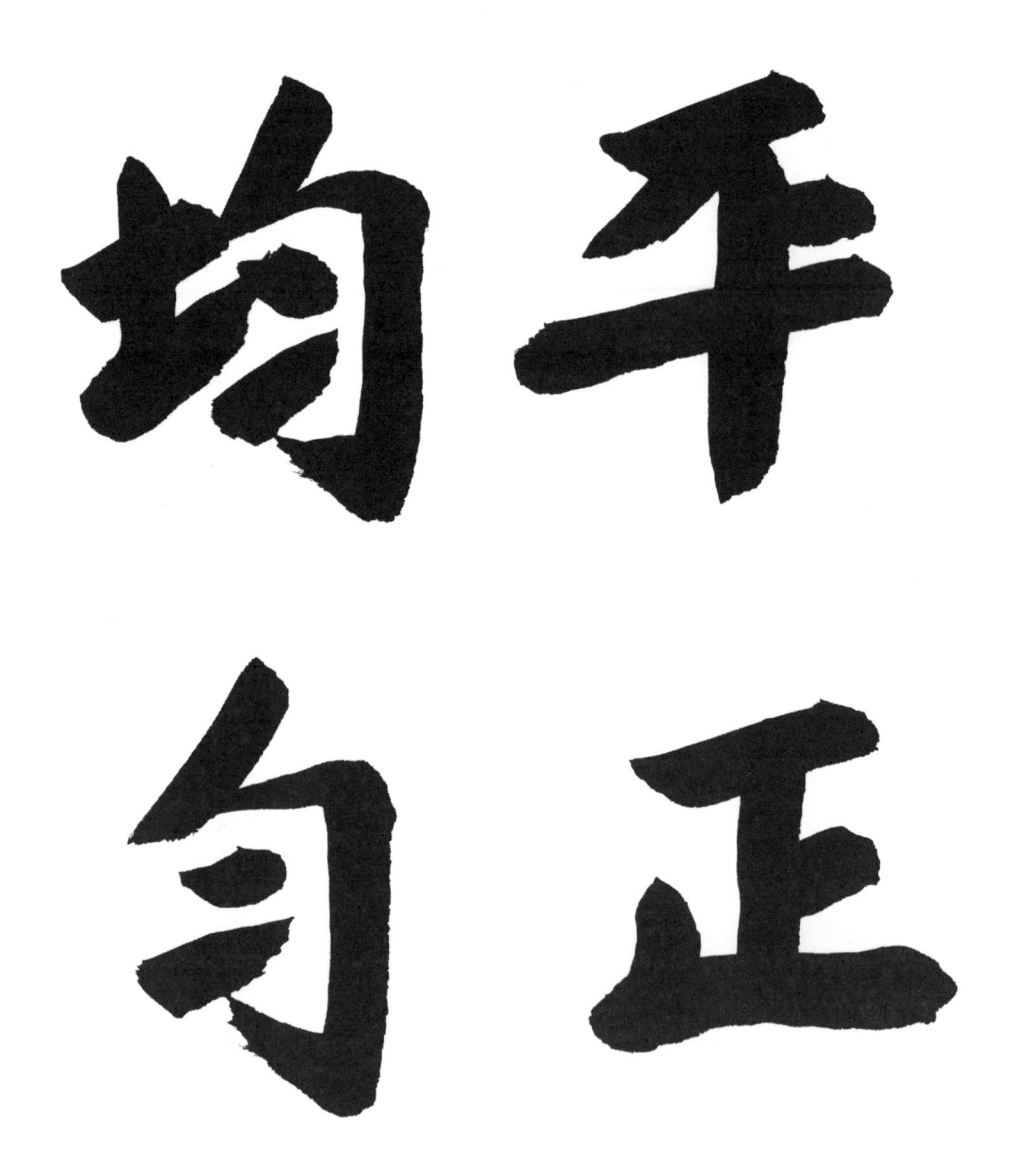

Unified   Balanced
Even   Upright

Cheng Man-Ch'ing says about these four basic concepts, a perfection in T'ai Chi Ch'uan can't be achieved without following them.

16. Master Chi's Ten Important Rules for Advanced Practice

1. Connect all the individual movements together into one movement.

2. Seek the unity of body and energy in the movement.

3. Move as lightly as possible.

4. Move naturally.

5. Always observe the Millstone Principle.

6. Not the movement of the arms, but the movement of the hips is essential.

7. When the arms are moved independently from the torso, one can't speak anymore of T'ai Chi Ch'uan.

8. Pay special attention to center equilibrium.

9. Develop natural breathing.

10. When practicing, concentrate on the lower Tan T'ien.

17. Two Aspects of the Forms: Practice and Application

In order to understand the forms better (short form and long form), they should be observed under both of the aspects "practice" and "application":

Practice. Practice of the forms serves all the developments attributed to T'ai Chi Ch'uan, especially the cultivation of the Chi. To create the best possible conditions for this, the movement sequences are placed together so that a clear and refined performance of the principles is possible. For that purpose, movements that are used fast and simultaneously in the application (self-defense) are performed slowly and one after another. The positions are connected by transitions that promote the Ch'i development through the continuous flow of movement. However, the essential core of the individual techniques is always retained.

Application. In self-defense, the positions are removed from their connections in the forms. The techniques contained within them are adjusted to the situation. The technique "Press," for instance, can be executed up, down, or forward. Steps and speed vary. The techniques can be combined in different ways.

18. Without Arms

The so-called "Without Arms" is an important basic rule in T'ai Chi Ch'uan. It states that the movement of the arms should always result out of the movement of the torso. Now this is even possible with rigidly held arms, synonymous with holding tight in the shoulders and elbows. The basic maxim "Without Arms" is only fulfilled when the shoulders and elbows are released, and the arms move as lightly as if one were without arms. Its compliance is of great significance for sinking the Ch'i and, therefore, for the Ch'i development. Yang Cheng-Fu says, without letting the shoulders and elbows relax, the Ch'i is held in the upper part of the body and can't sink. The Ch'i development remains correspondingly imperfect. The application of "Without Arms" is also important for self-defense. Dr. Chi explained it with the example of a ball.

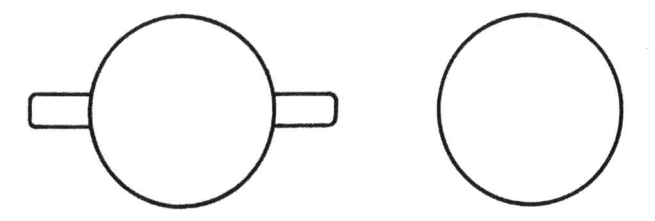

A ball with handles (stiff arms) can be much more easily seized than a ball without handles (relaxed arms). In the same way, in a quality T'ai Chi the movement sequences are presented so that they can be performed with relaxed shoulders and elbows.

19. Left Directs Left, Right Directs Right

This little-known basic maxim says that each half of the torso is followed in the movement by the limbs on that side. Through practicing this maxim attentively, we learn to better grasp the movements in their entirety and to perform in a refined manner the basic rules such as "Follow" and "Without Arms." Complying with it helps us to better distinguish between "Full" and "Empty," and it is particularly indispensable in the performance of Push Hands.

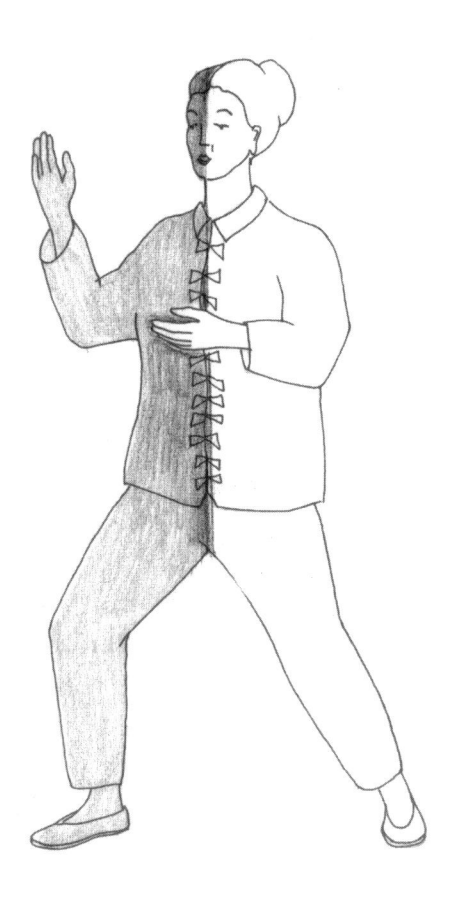

20. The Bow Step

Most of the movements are performed in the Bow Step; its correct performance is, therefore, of great importance.

Through the weight shift in the Bow Step and through the movements leading into and out of the Bow Step, softness and flexibility in the pelvic-abdominal area should be reached. This is of great importance for the deepening of the breathing and the use of the Ch'i. See Yang Cheng-Fu: "Only when the abdominal area is completely relaxed, can the Ch'i be set free in the sense of T'ai Chi Ch'uan."

The central maxim of T'ai Chi, "the hips lead the body in the movement" is also impossible to follow without an exceptional flexibility in the hip area.

In order to produce the desired effect, the Bow Step must be of a certain size. The basic rule is that it's longer than it's wide. The length should amount to one and one-half times the length of your foot, or somewhat less; the width should amount to the parallel standing position, where your feet are about one foot length apart (see diagram 1)

A relaxed movement in the correct Bow Step is usually not yet possible for beginners. In this case, it's recommended that you shorten the Bow Step. The relationship between its length and the width must still be guaranteed.

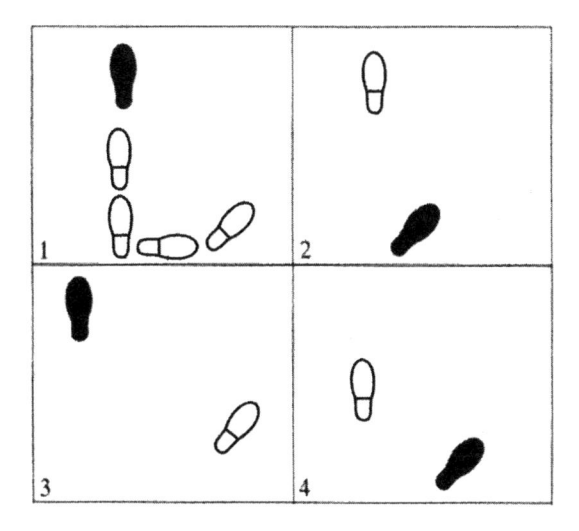

When the Bow Step is too narrow (diagram 2), too wide (diagram 3), or too short (diagram 4), the hip movement, in accord with the Millstone Principle (see the following) can't be correctly performed. In a too short Bow Step, space is missing for the movement from full to empty; in this way development and cultivation of the Ch'i can be decidedly affected.

With increasing softness and flexibility, the Bow Step "grows" and can eventually be used in the above-named size.

21. The Millstone Principle

In the hip area too, the movement should be even and flowing. When it's accompanied by a torso turn, it's comparable to the movement of a millstone ("Millstone Principle"). In order to fully develop the flexibility of the hip area and to arrive at a body movement really led by the hips, the Millstone Principle contains, next to this way of moving, the so-called "opening of the hip joints."[62] The following description is about the application of the Millstone Principle in the weight shift forward, into the Bow Step, and how it occurs, for instance, in Ward-Off Left, Brush Left Knee, and in the Single Whip.[63]

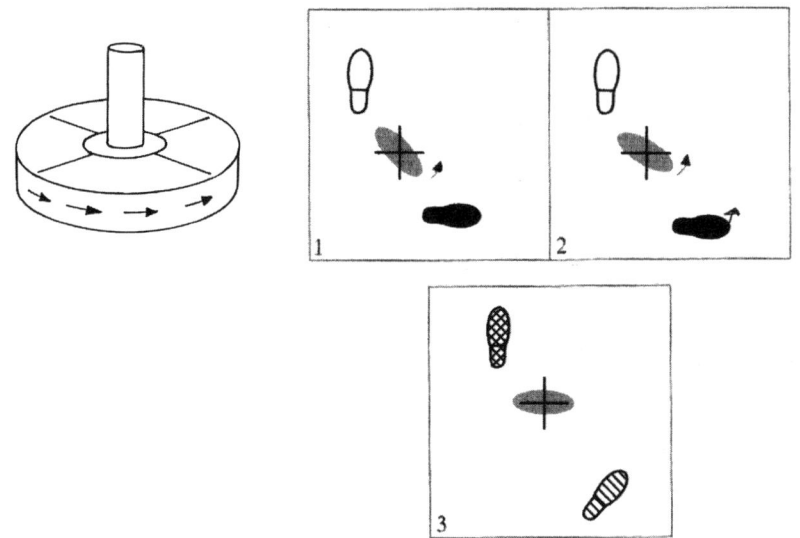

At the beginning of the weight shift, the torso turns somewhat to the left[64] (diagram 1), while the "full" back leg stands still. In this way, through turning away in the hip socket—the condyle stays still—the joint "opens." The following movement of the torso (diagrams 2–3) should then occur in the form of an arch so that the coccyx (tailbone), while moving, draws a small horizontal arch. The right foot is only turned in at the end of the movement.

Through this rather small unimportant-appearing movement sequence, the central principle of the rounded movement comes into use in the hip area, too. The Millstone Principle applies to all movements in the short form as well as the long form that occur with a turning movement of the torso! The correct performance of important techniques, such as the Rollback, for example, depends on the application of the Millstone Principle. When one wants to incorporate the Millstone Principle into one's practice, it's sensible to initially do so only on the horizontal. That means, at the end of the weight shift the center equilibrium shouldn't be performed, since connecting both the Millstone Principle and center equilibrium requires an established flexibility in the hip joints and

---
62 In the description of the form, the application of the Millstone Principle is noted.
63 For the use of the Millstone Principle in the weight shift backward, see the Millstone exercise on page 72.
64 When moving into the right Bow Step, the torso turns to the right.

leads into an even more demanding way of movement. Practicing the Millstone Principle develops, among other things, a more far-reaching centering. This can first be completely measured when one arrives at a relaxed even movement in the hip area, the entire practice method is refined, and one perceives the movement of the Ch'i.

22. The Millstone Exercise

1. Stand in the right Bow Step. Lift the arms (the lower arms as though lying on a board); 90 percent of the weight rests on the right foot.

2. Turn the torso somewhat to the left; the right leg remains unchanged (don't shift the weight); by turning left, the right hip joint is "opened."

3. Shift up to 70 percent of the weight onto the left foot. Turn the torso to the left; at the same, time the coccyx depicts a horizontal arch.[65]

4. Shift up to 90 percent of the weight onto the left foot. At the same time turn the torso to the right and "open" the left hip joint. The coccyx depicts a somewhat smaller arch than in 3.

5. Shift the weight to the front again; the torso turns to the left at the same time. The coccyx depicts a longer flat arch. Continue as in 2. In advanced practice, compliance with the Millstone Principle conveys the sensation of watching the movement of the body while resting in the middle.

   See Cheng Man-Ch'ing: "The millstone moves but the axis doesn't."[66]

It is advisable to practice the millstone exercise over a longer period of time, five minutes daily, in the right as well as in the left Bow Step.

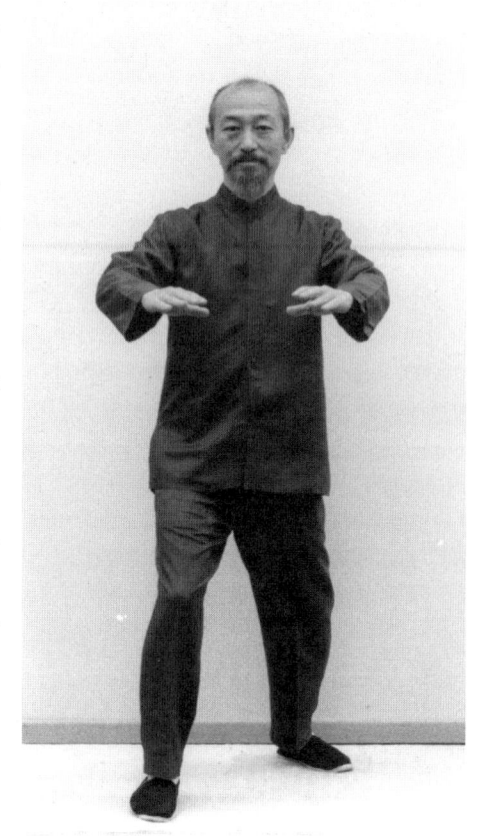

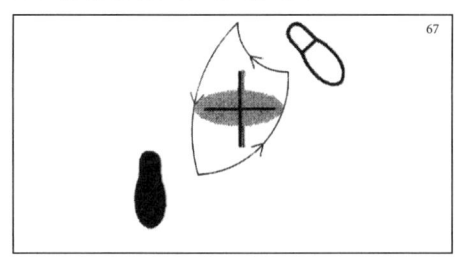

---

[65] As in the performance of Rollback. See Short Form position 5, photograph 2.
[66] Cheng Man-Ch'ing. *Thirteen Chapters on T'ai Chi Ch'uan*, page 102.
[67] The lines show the movements of the coccyx from the point of view of the practitioner. The picture of the millstone refers to each individual sequence of the movement. It doesn't describe a complete circular-shaped hip or coccyx movement.

23. Push Hands (Tui shou)

In this partner exercise, the positions that are combined under the name "Grasp the Sparrow's Tail"—Ward-Off, Rollback, Press, and Push—are removed from their connections in the form. They are then bound together so that they can be practiced selectively with a partner. Ward-Off, Rollback, Press, and Push are part of the thirteen basic positions. Their importance can be recognized by the frequency with which they are repeated in the short form and in the long form. The techniques connected with them are the foundations for self-defense in T'ai Chi Ch'uan. In Push Hands, the same principles apply as in the forms except for the speed. Push Hands is generally performed somewhat faster; the application of the techniques can also happen very rapidly.

The external motions of the partner exercise can be learned rather easily. In order to perform it in the T'ai Chi sense, a longer period of practicing is necessary. It's better to wait until the practitioner is more advanced to begin with an intensive training of Push Hands. Experience shows that when the practice of Push Hands is begun too early, one's existing movement habits tend to harden and stand in the way of improvement. This is especially true when there isn't a qualified teacher to guide the practice. Even when the practitioners rather rapidly acquire the abilities to bring each other out of the standing position, they are still far from the performance of quality T'ai Chi. Frequently they think they have developed a comprehensive knowledge about Push Hands after a few years and stop practicing.

In Push Hands, one should adjust to each different partner (beginner as well as advanced). To deepen what one has learned, it's helpful to practice regularly with the same partner.

The name commonly used for the partner in T'ai Chi, "player," clearly demonstrates the spirit in which working together on the principles should take place.[68]

The principles without arms, no force, lightness, let go and the clear differentiation between "full" and "empty" need to receive special attention for a long time. Particularly in Push Hands, there is a great temptation to ignore these important principles.

In Push Hands, it's a question of learning a refined application of the techniques Ward-Off, Rollback, Press, and Push. The widespread practice in Push Hands of shoving each other off balance through a strong pulling and pushing without paying any attention to these techniques is not the idea of the exercise. It is also advisable to first identify one's own mistakes and then the ones of the partner. In T'ai Chi Ch'uan, we say that our partner is our "mirror." We only experience his or her "hardness" as disturbing, for example, because we ourselves are not yet "soft" enough.

---

[68] At the end of practicing one often compliments one's partner by saying, "Thank you, you play very well."

The Application of the Various Chin in Push Hands

When the partners are advanced, the various Chin (see page 51) can be increasingly applied in the practice of Push Hands. The individual Chin are the expression of the developed Ch'i, which is now felt as "condensed" or "tenacious" energy.[69] The Nien Chin (sticking energy), for instance, leads to an intensive awareness of the intentions of the opponent. It permits a yielding without losing contact with the partner. The Ting Chin (hearing or understanding energy) lets us find the partner's center of gravity and enables us to bring him out of balance.

Uprooting

The most well-known application of tenacious energy used in Push Hands in the techniques of Ward-Off, Press, and Push is uprooting. T'i Chin (uprooting energy) is employed here. Without effort, the partner should be lifted from the floor, and he is thrown several meters. To identify if it has been a true uprooting, Tung Ying Chieh suggests paying attention that the performer remains "perfectly at ease" while using the energy.[70]

Before the use of energy in uprooting, the weight is usually shifted backward. A slight bending of the knees together with letting go and sinking results in the energy accumulating in the area of the lower Tan T'ien and the back foot. Through a small even movement of the body, starting from the foot, the energy is mobilized and directed to the partner so that he is "uprooted." The posture of the spinal column and especially the lower back (sacrum) receives special importance in setting the energy free.

The movement sequence described usually occurs very rapidly. In *The Song of Push Hands,* it says: "Opening and closing occur in a moment."

When a strong force is first directed against us, it can not only be deflected but also used (borrowing energy) by guiding it to the back foot. It supports the accumulation of the Ch'i there and afterward can be directed back to the partner. The practice of Push Hands leads to an interesting experience in this connection. The energy moving between the practitioners can't be divided as "mine" or "yours," but rather is experienced as one energy of which both have a share.

For the use of tenacious energy in uprooting, observe the following important points that we learned from Dr. Chi.

1. The Distance

The distance to the partner must be exactly right. If it is too large, the energy sent out disperses. If it is too small, one can't correctly set the energy free.

---

[69] Dr. Chi described some of the results that a highly developed tenacious energy brings with it: "The practitioner no longer has two arms but rather many arms.... His hand sticks to his partner as though it were glued to him.... His body appears to be filled with a gaseous substance that gives him elasticity, an attacking strength for protection through immediate natural reactions."

[70] A good example of a complete uprooting is shown by Cheng Man-Ch'ing in the book by Cheng Man-Ch'ing and Robert W. Smith, *T'ai Chi: The "Supreme Ultimate" Exercise for Health, Sport, and Self-Defense* (pages 88–89).

2. The Angle

The energy must be directed at the partner in the correct angle. When the partner leans himself to the side or is already in a position from which he can no longer escape, it is especially easy to find his center of gravity.

3. The Time

The use of energy must come at the right time: the attack of the partner has just ended and a new one hasn't begun yet or when he is just pulling back.

4. The Opportunity

When the timing, distance, and angle are right, the necessary prerequisites exist for setting energy free.

5. Calmness

During the use of energy, the practitioner should remain perfectly calm.

6. Accumulating the Energy before Use

The classical texts tell us to "store the energy before you use it." The accumulation of energy is like drawing a bowstring before releasing an arrow. When one follows this example, one can easily set energy free.

7. Unity

At the last moment before the energy is set free, the legs and hips must be brought into the correct position so that a unified movement of the entire body is possible, starting at the feet. (See the classical texts: "The energy is rooted in the feet, flows through the legs, is directed by the hips, and is expressed through the hands.")

8. Distinction between "Full" and "Empty"

In the use of energy, only one arm can be "full."

9. The Significance of the Arms

When an arm moves alone, the energy can't be sent out in the T'ai Chi Ch'uan sense. Only from the unity of body, mind, and Ch'i in the movement can our partner be uprooted by the rules of T'ai Chi.

10. The Direction

The energy should be sent out with complete concentration in one direction.

11. Attentive Observation of the Partner

During the entire sequence described, all the possible movements of the partner must be observed and taken into account.

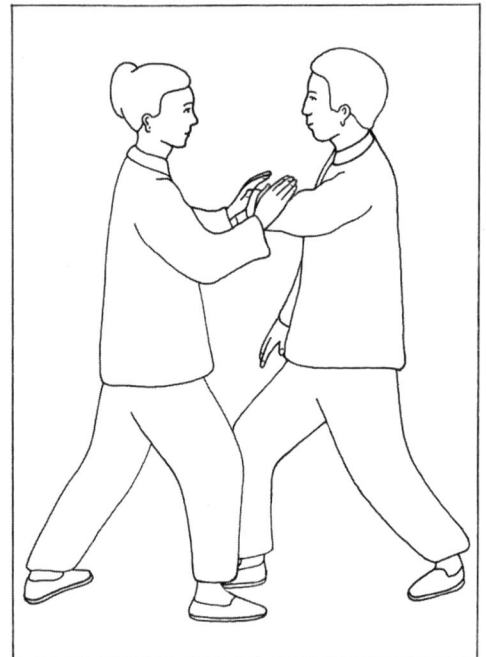

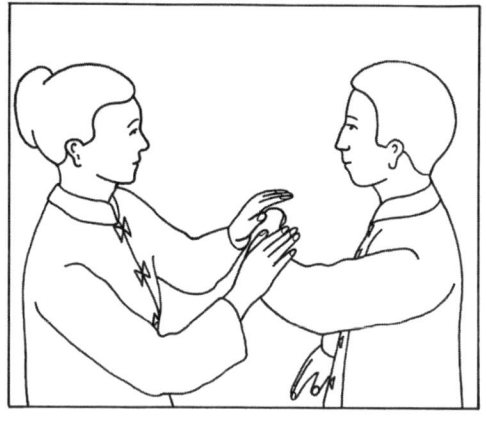

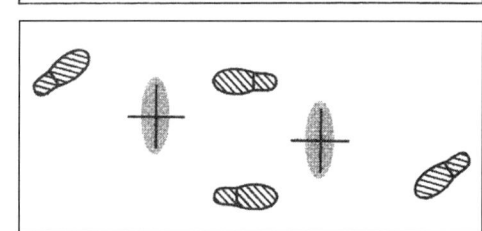

PUSH HANDS

Diagrams 1 and 1a

Beginning position: Both partners (A and B) stand opposite each other in the right Bow Step. B lifts his left arm (Ward-Off), palm of the hand turned to the body. A lifts both arms (Push), both palms of the hands lightly touch the left lower arm of B, the left hand lies on the left wrist of B.

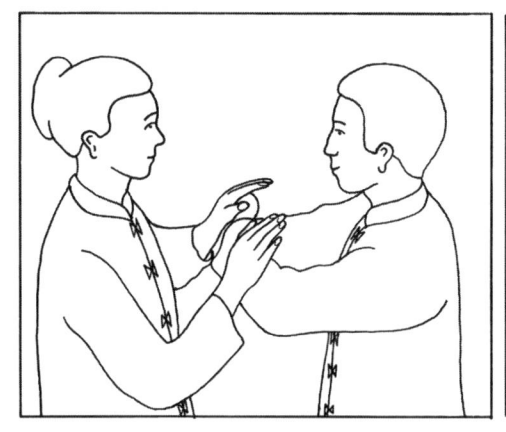

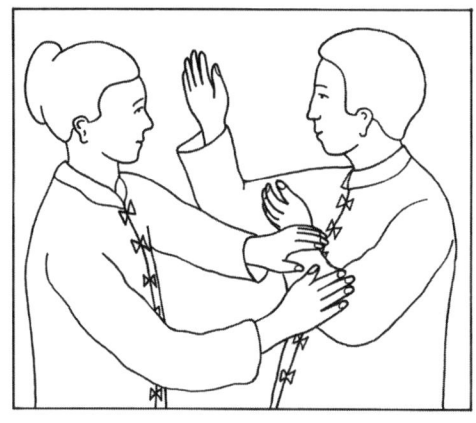

Diagrams 2 and 3

A shifts up to 70 percent of her weight onto the right foot and performs the "Push." B neutralizes A through yielding and performs the "Rollback": He turns his torso (Millstone Principle) to the left and shifts 70 percent of his weight onto the back foot. In the beginning of the movement, he has already raised his right arm (diagram 2) and touches somewhat below his elbow, the left arm of A (also somewhat below the elbow).* Accompanying the torso turn and the weight shift, he angles his arm for the "Rollback."

A follows B after the performance of "Push" by turning her torso somewhat to the right.

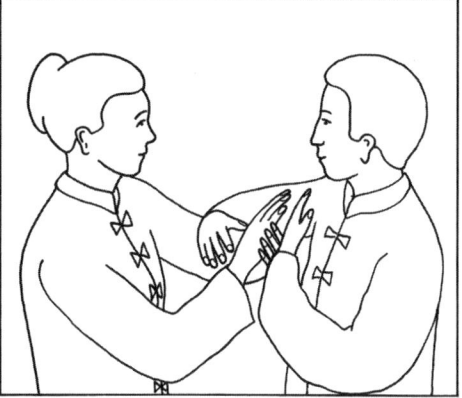

Diagram 4

A turns her torso to the left until her front side faces forward, shifts up to 90 percent of her weight onto the front foot, and performs "Press" directly forward to B's breastbone: First she turns the left hand counterclockwise until the back of her hand touches B's left wrist and then places her right hand lightly on the wrist of his left hand.

B yields and neutralizes A by turning his torso right and shifting up to 90 percent of his weight onto the back foot. Simultaneously, he sinks his right arm (lower arm and hand as a unit) in front of his body, and places his hand (palm) lightly on the right wrist of A.†

After the performance of "Press," A follows B by turning her torso somewhat left.

---
* In order to "control" A's elbows.
† In order to "control" A's wrist.

Diagram 5

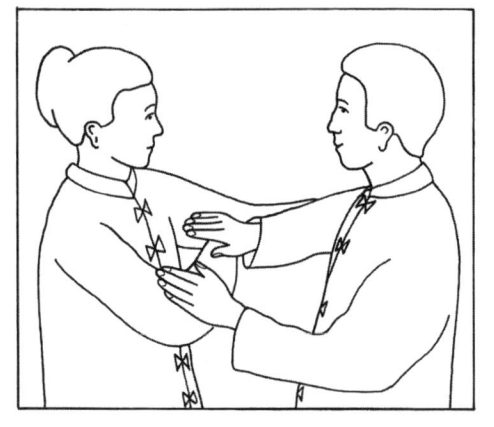

B prepares to "Push."* He turns his torso somewhat farther to the right and bends his knee (release in the groin area, Center Equilibrium). At the same time, he brings his right arm under A's left arm, directs his hand then, in an arch moving clockwise, to A's lower arm, and lightly places it on her right wrist (Push). Simultaneously, he also lowers his left arm (relax in the elbows), and places the left hand (palm) on A's lower arm (Push).

During B's preparation of the "Push," A had already reacted by preparing the "Rollback." Accompanying the release in the groin area of her front leg, she lifts her left arm following a clockwise arch on the right side of B's body and touches his arm below the elbow (Rollback).† Simultaneously, she lowers the right arm in front of her body and turns it clockwise (hand and lower arm as a unit) (Rollback).††

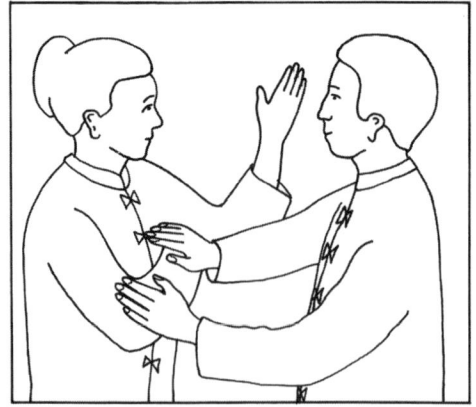

Diagram 6

B performs "Push." While doing this, he first turns his torso to the left until his front side faces forward. A neutralizes B through yielding and performs "Rollback": She turns her torso (Millstone Principle) to the right and shifts 70 percent of her weight onto the back foot. Accompanying her torso turn and weight shift, she angles her arm for "Rollback."

After the performance of "Push," B follows A by turning his torso somewhat to the left.

---

*Yielding and the preparation for pushing are a smooth transition: "Yielding is attacking."
† In order to "control" B's elbows.
†† So that B's hands can be correctly placed on A's lower arm.

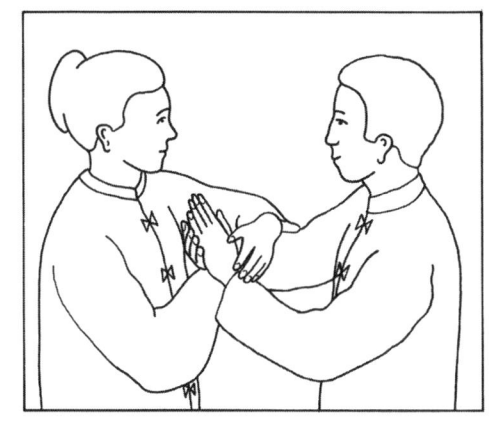

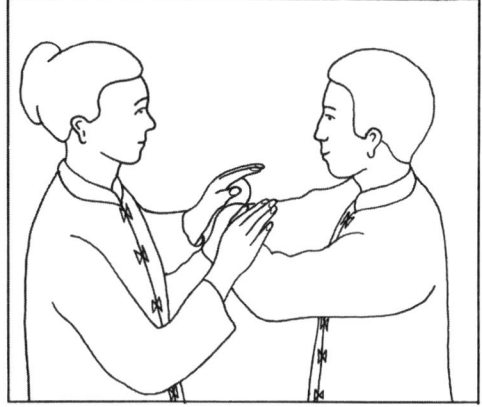

Diagram 7

B turns his torso to the right until his front side faces front and then performs "Press" directly forward to A's breastbone; in addition, he first turns his right hand clockwise until the back of his hand touches A's right wrist and then places his left hand lightly on the lower inside palm of his right hand.

A yields and neutralizes B by turning her torso to the left, and at the same time shifts up to 90 percent of her weight onto her back foot. Simultaneously, she lowers her left arm (lower arm and hand as a unit) in front of her body and places her hand (palm) lightly on B's wrist.

Diagram 8

A prepares to "Push": She turns her torso somewhat further to the left and bends her knee (release in the groin area, Center Equilibrium). While doing so, she brings her left arm under B's right arm, guides her hand following a clockwise arch to B's lower arm and places it lightly on his left wrist (Push). Simultaneously, she also lowers her right arm (release in the elbows) and places the right hand (palm) on B's lower-arm (Push).

During the preparation of the "Push," B had already reacted by preparing the "Rollback." Accompanying the release in the groin area of his front leg, he lifts his right arm, following a counterclockwise arch on the left side of A's body and touches her left arm below the elbow (Rollback); simultaneously, he lowers the left arm in front of the body and turns it (hand and lower arm as a unit) counterclockwise (Rollback).*

Next, A performs "Push" in sequence. Continue as above.

---

* So that A's hands can be correctly placed on B's lower arm.

24. The Short Form

The short form of the Yang-style was developed by Professor Cheng Man-Ch'ing. Its basis is the long form of his teacher Yang Cheng-Fu. It contains thirty-seven positions (with repetitions, sixty-four). Compared with Yang Cheng-Fu's long form, which contains fifty-three positions (with repetitions, 140), it becomes clear that Cheng Man-Ch'ing has taken out not only positions but mainly repetitions. He retained the sequence of the positions. When one knows the long form of his teacher, one recognizes that the positions removed were sixteen of those that are particularly demanding to perform, such as "Needle at Sea Bottom," "High Pat on Horse," "Hit the Tiger Left and Right," and so on. Moreover, Cheng Man-Ch'ing doesn't divide the second and third parts through the repetition of the sequence (Withdraw and Push; Cross Hands).

In the performance too, the short form is different than the long form. The movements in the short form are less expansive, and the arms are usually held lower, which is helpful for beginners. Cheng Man-Ch'ing also simplified the procedure of the weight shift. While in the long form the changes in direction are often taken on the weight-carrying foot, he shifts the weight back before he changes the direction.

Cheng Man-Ch'ing himself described his short form as "simplified." With the simplification of the normally difficult to learn traditional classical T'ai Chi, it became accessible to a wider range of people. In spite of these and other simplifications that Cheng Man-Ch'ing introduced, the short form contains all the essential elements of a quality T'ai Chi Ch'uan, including the thirteen basic positions.

The short form presented in this book is based on the short form we learned from Dr. Chi. Since Professor Cheng Man-Ch'ing as well as his students continued to modify details in the short form, various versions exist.[71] These changes appear, for example, in the use of different self-defense techniques in individual positions. Some teachers have also included long form positions (William Chen–style).

The short form has three parts. The transitions between the positions are counted as part of the following position.

Performing the short form usually takes six to eight minutes.

---

[71] In Taipei, Professor Cheng Man-Ch'ing taught both the short form as well as the long form. He taught them both with the characteristics we now know as his special imprint on T'ai Chi. In the United States, he chose to teach only the short form.

25. Remarks about Practicing

1. Knee

Deep bending of the knees isn't recommended for beginners. It leads to excessive stress on the knee joints and encourages incorrect posture that might have an impairing effect. Only after increased practice should the movements gradually be performed somewhat lower.

2. Bow Step

Pay attention not to take a Bow Step that is both too wide and too short. If you do this, you will shift the weight sideways instead of back and forth. This blocks the lively and directed movement.

3. Eyes

At the end of a position, the eyes look straight ahead.[72] In the transitions, your eyes should follow the movement. The gaze shouldn't be fixed.

4. Surroundings

In the first years of practicing, one is often distracted by things or movement in one's surroundings. When this ceases to occur, the practitioner has achieved considerable progress.

5. Inner Smile

The image of an "inner smile" helps to relax the face and sink the Ch'i.

6. Sink

Particular attention should be paid to the light, relaxed, and even performance of all the necessary movements needed for sinking the Ch'i, such as the gradual bending of the knees and the lowering of the arms into the standing hand (see page 83).

7. Lifting and Sinking the Arms and Legs

The principle of the unity of the body in the movement requires that lifting an arm goes with a light stretching of the knee, and that sinking an arm goes with a light bending of the knee (for example, the movements that lead into and out of "Stork Spreads Wings"). The same applies to the lifting and sinking of the legs before and after the kicks.

---

[72] In the partner exercise, the attention is on the partner.

8. "When one is up, one shouldn't forget down; when one is in front, one shouldn't forget the back."

This basic maxim is closely linked to the unity of the body in movement. In the weight shift in the Bow Step, for example, our attention should be on the "filling" of one foot as well as on "emptying" the other one and comprehending the movement in its entirety.

9. Coordinated Movement

This principle requires that all the individual movements of the different parts of the body that lead into a position are begun and ended simultaneously. That means that the movement of the torso and the individual limbs usually have different speeds. (In the position "Stork Spreads Wings," for example, a very small movement in the hip area must be coordinated with a wide-reaching movement of the right arm).

10. Lively, Directed Movement

Particular attention should be paid that the movement is lively and directed. Directing the movement to the part of the body that comes into contact with the opponent in each position—hand, fist, elbow, foot, and so on—substantially supports the liveliness of the movement.

11. Conscious Ch'i Development

Through the image of pulling a silken thread from a cocoon, the Ch'i development through movement is considerably reinforced (see page 27).

12. Perception of Ch'i

Practitioners often react to their first perception of the Ch'i with astonishment, but it gradually becomes a trusted and welcomed companion in practicing. It's an indication that we are on the right path in our development.

13. Breathing

T'ai Chi is in its structure already a breathing exercise. The cultivation of extensive softness and flexibility of the entire body creates the best conditions for the deepening of respiration. In this way, chest breathing—which occurs in the majority of people—deepens through exercising into abdominal breathing in a natural way. Abdominal breathing, which is also called "natural breathing," is extremely beneficial for the Ch'i development!

A coordination of breathing with movement should first be attempted when the movement sequences have been well learned. Knowledge should also be available about where the phases of breathing in (collecting) and breathing out (directing) are located in the flow of the form.

Beginners should allow breathing to occur by itself. Experience shows that breathing regulates itself to the movement: breathing in when shifting backward, and breathing out when shifting forward.

14. The T'ai Chi Hand

The concept "T'ai Chi hand" includes the position of the fingers as well as the position of the hand in relation to the lower arm.

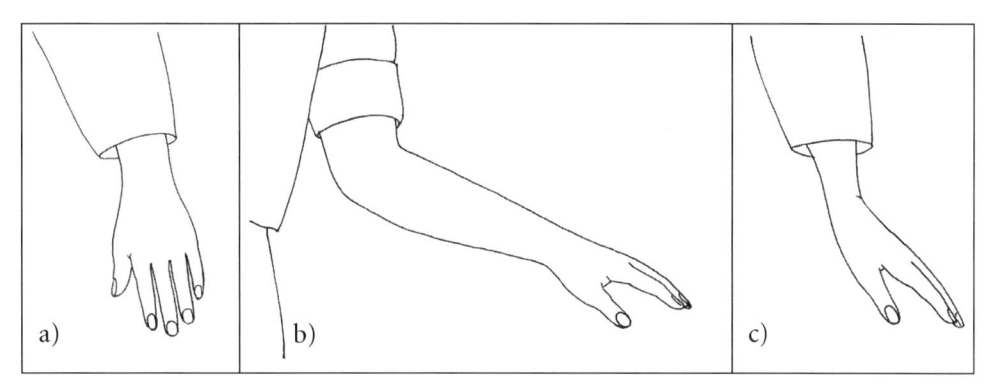

a) The fingers are slightly opened.
b) The lower arm and the back of the hand form an almost straight, but slightly rounded, line. This unit remains during the movement: the lower arm and hand are raised and lowered, as well as turned from the elbow joint. The T'ai Chi hand is used in all movements of the arm except in the "standing hand," the "fist," and the "bird's head" (see Single Whip page 103).

15. The Standing Hand [73]

Toward the end of many positions, the light and relaxed standing hand position, is taken. In it, the back of the hand and the lower arm form an angle of about 135 degrees, which supports the direction of energy outward. See the classical texts: "The energy is expressed through the hands."

---

[73] A specific feature of Cheng Man-Ch'ing's personal performance was that he retained the T'ai Chi hand, which he called the "beautiful lady's hand," during the entire performance of the form except the hand positions "fist" and "bird's head." This was only in connection with practicing the form. In the application of self-defense, he also used the standing hand.

16. The Principle of the Unity of Movement

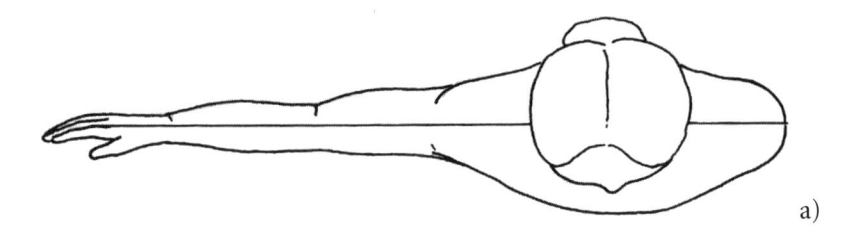

a) When lifting an arm backward, the imaginary line extending between the shoulders shouldn't be exceeded.

b) The active (attacking) arm shouldn't move outside the dark lines in this diagram. In this way, the energy movement fills the arm fully.

c) The torso shouldn't go beyond the line drawn to the heels.

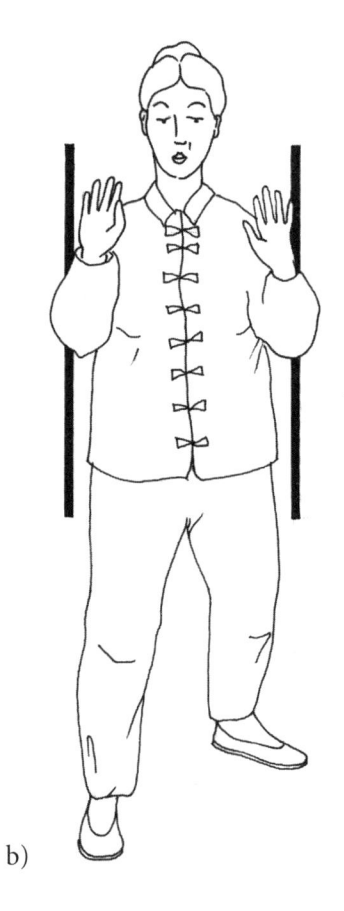

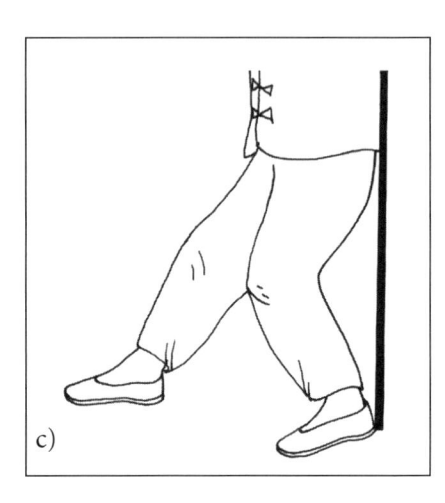

17. The Hips and Center Equilibrium

In all the movements, the hips should be kept on a horizontal line.

The performance of center equilibrium takes place in the groin fold toward the end of the weight shift, focusing on the middle of the upper thigh. The groin fold is the crease that appears when you relax in the area between the upper thigh and the torso.

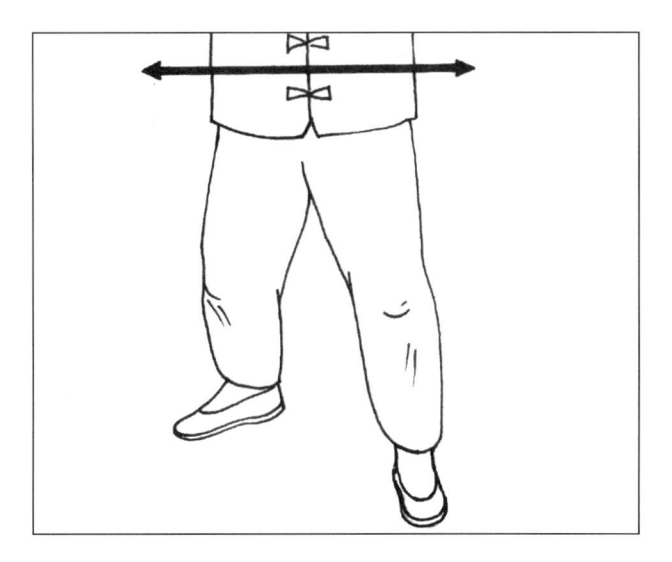

18. Lifting the Legs

The lifting of the legs should proceed as relaxed as possible. Even at the end of the positions, legs as well as arms shouldn't be completely stretched out.

19. Mistakes

The knees hang down, causing the Bow Step to lose the necessary tension. The unified and lively movement is considerably affected. A clear balance between Heaven Ch'i and Earth Ch'i is difficult to achieve.

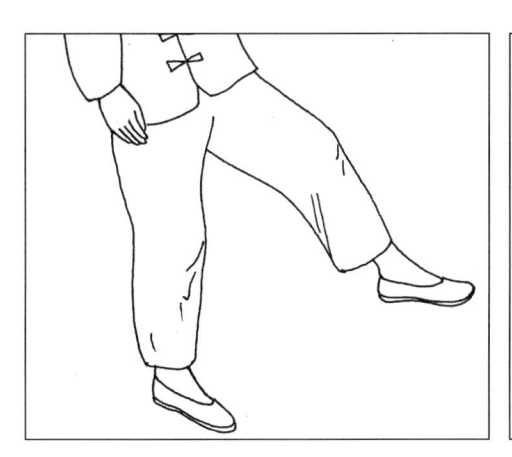

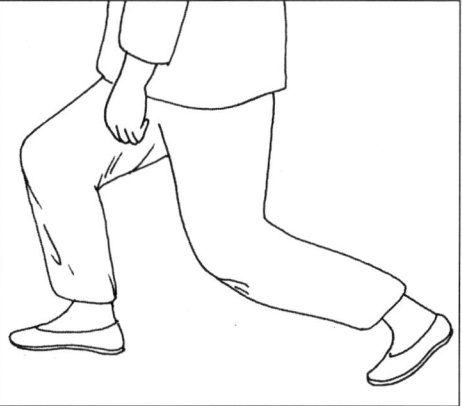

26. Important Questions to Ask Yourself When Correcting Your Own Practice

1. Is the movement experienced as pleasant, light, and natural?

2. Are the steps correctly taken: Bow Step, Parallel Stance, Step of the Fishing Horse, and T-Step?

3. Do the arms and legs follow the movement of the torso (hips)?

4. Is the erect, upright posture of the spinal column maintained during the changes in direction and the steps?

5. Are the turning movements in the hip area even and flowing?

6. Are the joints moved evenly and smoothly?

7. Are the movements rounded, following the shape of an arch?

8. Have you relaxed as much as possible (face, hands, shoulders)?

9. Is the shifting backward performed with the same level of attention as shifting forward?

10. Does the movement impulse come from the feet?

11. Is the breathing deep, calm, fine, and inaudible?

12. Are you concentrating on the lower Tan T'ien or using complete attentiveness during the entire course of the movement?

13. Are "full and empty," "open and close," "sink," and "center equilibrium" used?

27. Advice on Learning the Short Form

The text below refers to what is being depicted in the corresponding picture. When first learning the sequence of the movements, it is recommended that practitioners begin to include the arm movements only after clarity has been reached about the movements of the torso and the legs.

In explaining the photos that follow, we will begin by describing the torso movement, following the principle that "the hips direct the body in the movement." The individual movements described with every photo begin and end simultaneously.

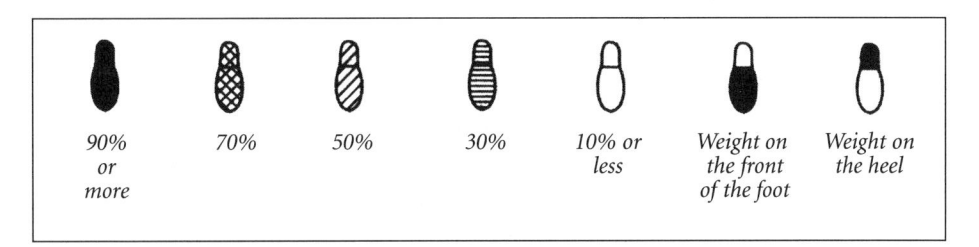

| 90% or more | 70% | 50% | 30% | 10% or less | Weight on the front of the foot | Weight on the heel |

The foot diagrams under the photographs show the appropriate distribution of weight and the position of the feet at that particular point. As you can see in the following text and diagrams about steps, the position of the feet are either directed to the main compass points (N, S, E, W) or the points between them (NE, NW, SW, SE), which are also called 45 degrees or diagonal. A number of positions differ slightly from this standard. In certain techniques, one foot or both feet can be placed at 30 degrees. This would be 30 degrees to either the left or the right of the closest main compass point.

The hip diagrams are thought of as an additional aid to make the sequence of the movement clearer. They show the particular position of the torso. The torso is invariably moved as a unit from the hips. When a torso turn is mentioned, it normally means that the head turns, too. There are only a few places where the head and torso movements don't occur together. (Following an old maxim, the head should not move independently from the torso, but in some positions the torso may be moved independently from the head.)

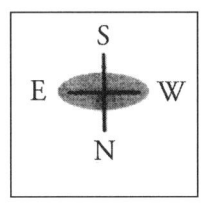

The arrows show the direction of the movement sequences leading into the next photograph. The movements of the limbs following an arch can best be understood from them.

The basic steps are presented in the following table.

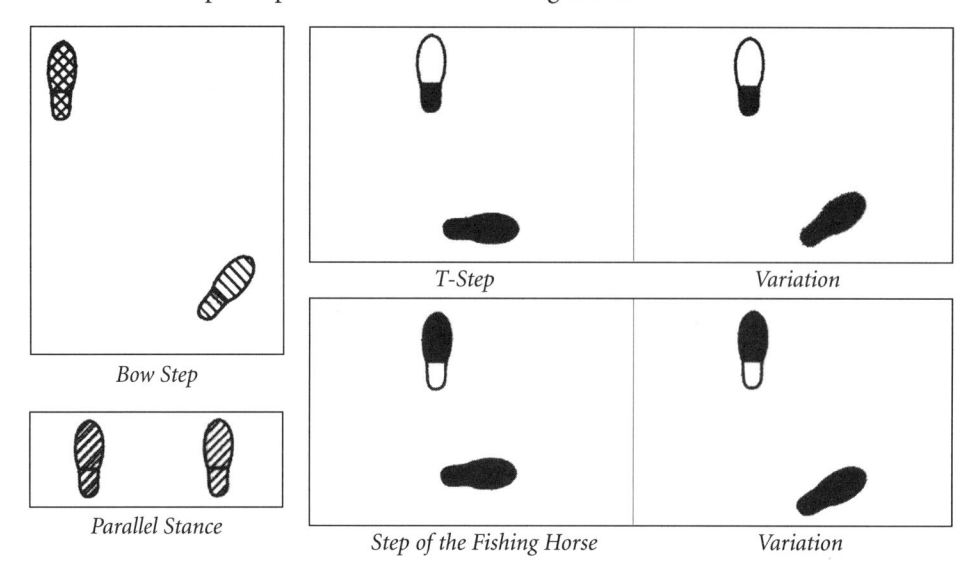

Bow Step	T-Step	Variation
Parallel Stance	Step of the Fishing Horse	Variation

Bow Step: It is advisable for beginners to perform the torso turning in the Bow Step as follows: first shift most of the body weight onto the front foot, then turn, as a unit, the torso, leg, and foot on the heel. When the form has been learned well, a different variation should be practiced: at the start of the weight shift, begin already turning the torso and leg on the heel as a unit; the torso turn and weight shift occur simultaneously.[74] In advanced practice, with increasing softness and flexibility, the weight shift and the torso turn should follow the Millstone Principle (see page 70).

Step of the Fishing Horse: In the Step of the Fishing Horse you have the weight of your body on the back leg, and your front leg is lifted so that only the front part of the foot touches the ground. (Horses standing in shallow water have the habit of repeatedly lifting one front leg out of the water and putting it down again.)

Let go (release), sink; and the Millstone Principle are only included in the description where it appears to be especially important to call attention to them again. Normally, they should be used as described earlier.

To help in understanding the direction of the movements, we use the points of the compass (N, S, E, W, SW, NE, NWW, SEE, and so on). Independent of the actual points of the compass, the direction in which one begins the exercise is called North.[75]

---

[74] In most of the T'ai Chi directions, one of these two variations is used.
[75] In addition to using the compass for orientation, the direction of the dial of a clock is commonly used.

Due to the angles of some of the photographs, the feet, torso, or arms might be difficult to recognize. In case of doubt, refer to the descriptions and diagrams.
Note: During the repetition of positions, the transitions vary according to the point of departure.

28. List of the Positions—Short Form

Part 1

1. Preparation
2. Beginning (Awaken the Ch'i)
3. Grasp the Sparrow's Tail—Ward-Off, Left
4. Grasp the Sparrow's Tail—Ward-Off, Right
5. Grasp the Sparrow's Tail—Rollback
6. Grasp the Sparrow's Tail—Press
7. Grasp the Sparrow's Tail—Push
8. Single Whip
9. Lift Hands
10. Shoulder Push (Lean Forward)
11. Stork Spreads Wings
12. Brush Left Knee—Twist Step
13. Play the Lute
    Brush Left Knee—Twist Step (12)
14. Step Forward, Deflect Downward, Parry, and Punch
15. Withdraw and Push
16. Cross Hands

Part 2

17. Embrace Tiger and Return to Mountain
    Grasp the Sparrow's Tail—
    Rollback (5)
    Grasp the Sparrow's Tail—Press (6)
    Grasp the Sparrow's Tail—Push (7)
    Single Whip (8)
18. Fist under Elbow
19. Step Back and Repulse Monkey, Right
20. Step Back and Repulse Monkey, Left
    Step Back and Repulse Monkey, Right (19)
21. Diagonal Flying
22. Wave Hands in Clouds, Left
23. Wave Hands in Clouds, Right
    Wave Hands in Clouds, Left (22)
    Wave Hands in Clouds, Right (23)
    Wave Hands in Clouds, Left (22)
    Single Whip (8)
24. Squatting Single Whip
25. Golden Cock Stands on One Leg, Right
26. Golden Cock Stands on One Leg, Left
27. Separate Right Foot
28. Separate Left Foot
29. Turn and Kick with Left Heel
    Brush Left Knee—Twist Step (12)
30. Brush Right Knee—Twist Step
31. Step Forward and Strike with Fist
    Grasp the Sparrow's Tail—
    Ward-Off, Right (4)
    Grasp the Sparrow's Tail—
    Rollback (5)
    Grasp the Sparrow's Tail—
    Press (6)
    Grasp the Sparrow's Tail—
    Push (7)
    Single Whip (8)

Part 3

32. Fair Lady Works at Shuttle, Left
33. Fair Lady Works at Shuttle, Right
    Fair Lady Works at Shuttle, Left (32)
    Fair Lady Works at Shuttle, Right (33)
    Grasp the Sparrow's Tail—
    Ward-Off, Left (3)
    Grasp the Sparrow's Tail—
    Ward-Off, Right (4)
    Grasp the Sparrow's Tail—
    Rollback (5)
    Grasp the Sparrow's Tail—Press (6)
    Grasp the Sparrow's Tail—Push (7)
    Single Whip (8)
    Squatting Single Whip (24)
34. Step Forward to Seven Stars
35. Step Back and Ride Tiger
36. Turn and Sweep Over Lotus with Leg
37. Bend Bow and Shoot Tiger
    Step Forward, Deflect Downward
    Parry, and Punch (14)
    Withdraw and Push (15)
    Cross Hands (16)
    Conclusion

29. The Short Form

Part 1. Preparation

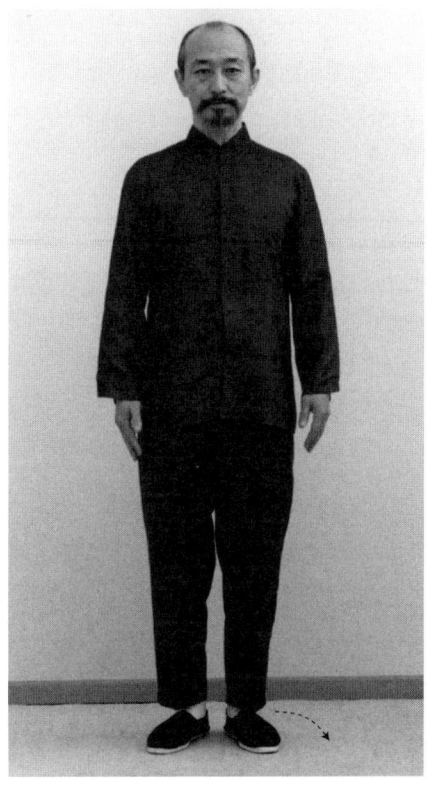

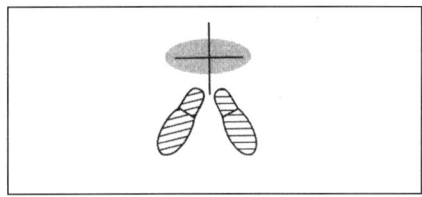

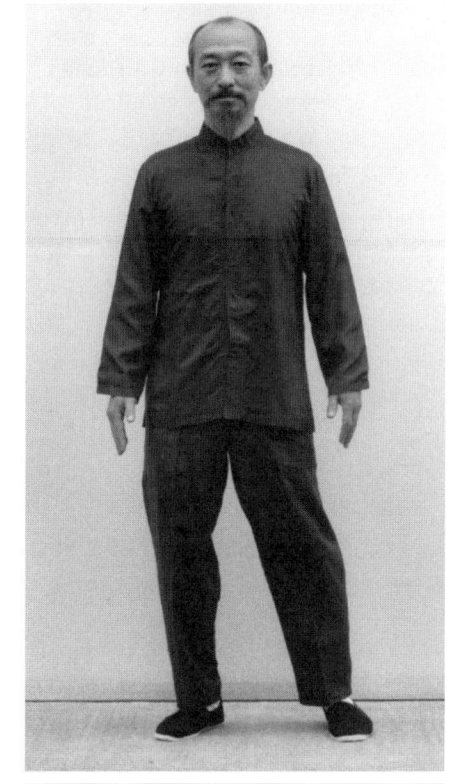

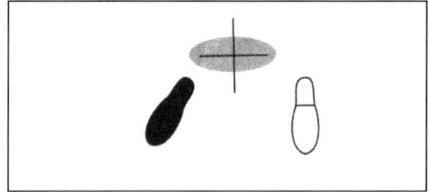

1. The heels are together. The weight is evenly distributed on both feet. The knees are slightly bent. The spine is held upright. The arms hang relaxed. The palms of the hands are turned toward the thighs (T'ai Chi hand). You face North.

Not shown: Shift the weight onto the right foot by bending the right knee. At the same time, lift the heel of the left foot.

2. Place the left leg about one foot length to the left side, placing the inner edge of the foot down first (Parallel Stance). The toes point N.

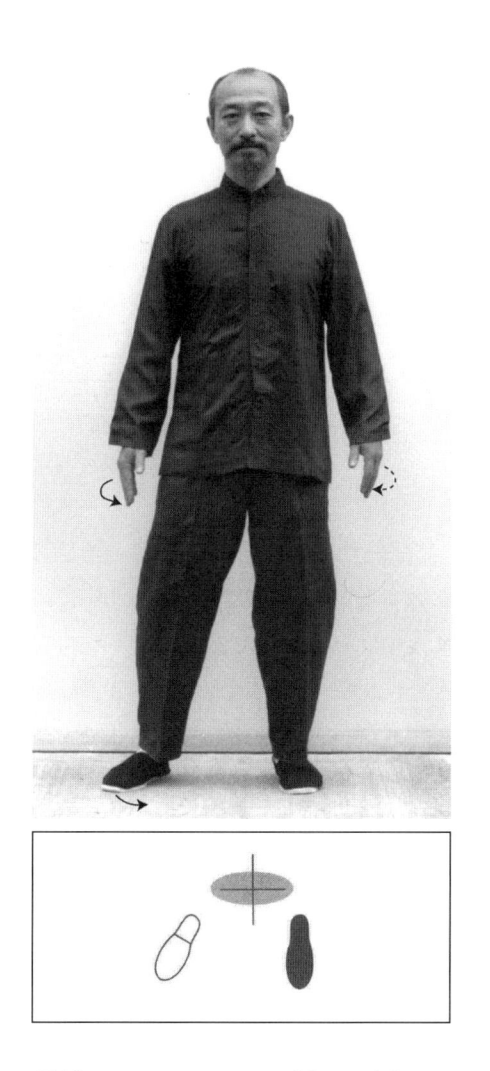

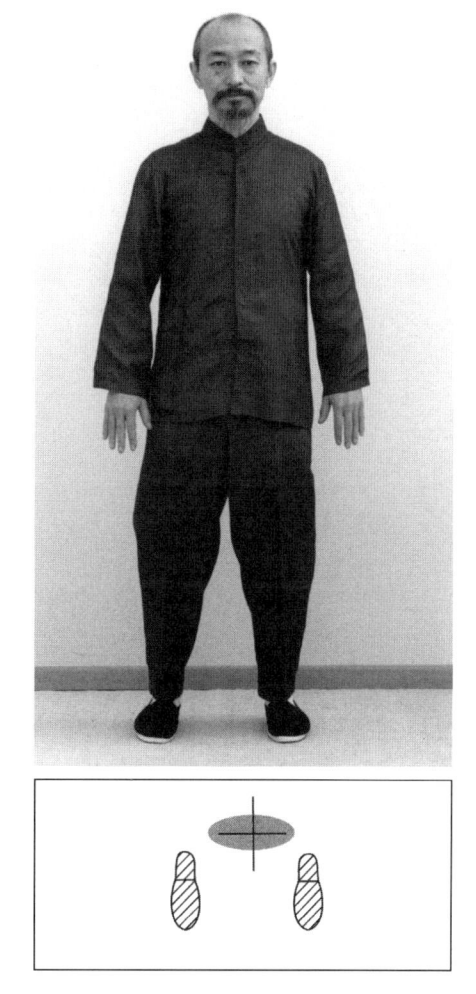

3. Shift up to 90 percent of the weight onto the left foot. Don't turn the torso!

4. Through a slight turning of the torso to the left, turn the right foot on the heel until it is parallel to the left foot. At the same time, begin small circles to the front with both arms. Note: The movement of the arms follows the elbow joints; the lower arm and hand move as one unit (T'ai Chi hand).

Then shift up to 50 percent of the weight onto the right foot. At the same time, complete the circular movement of the arms. Toward the end of the movement, indicate the position "standing hand" (release, sink).

2. Beginning (Awaken the Ch'i)

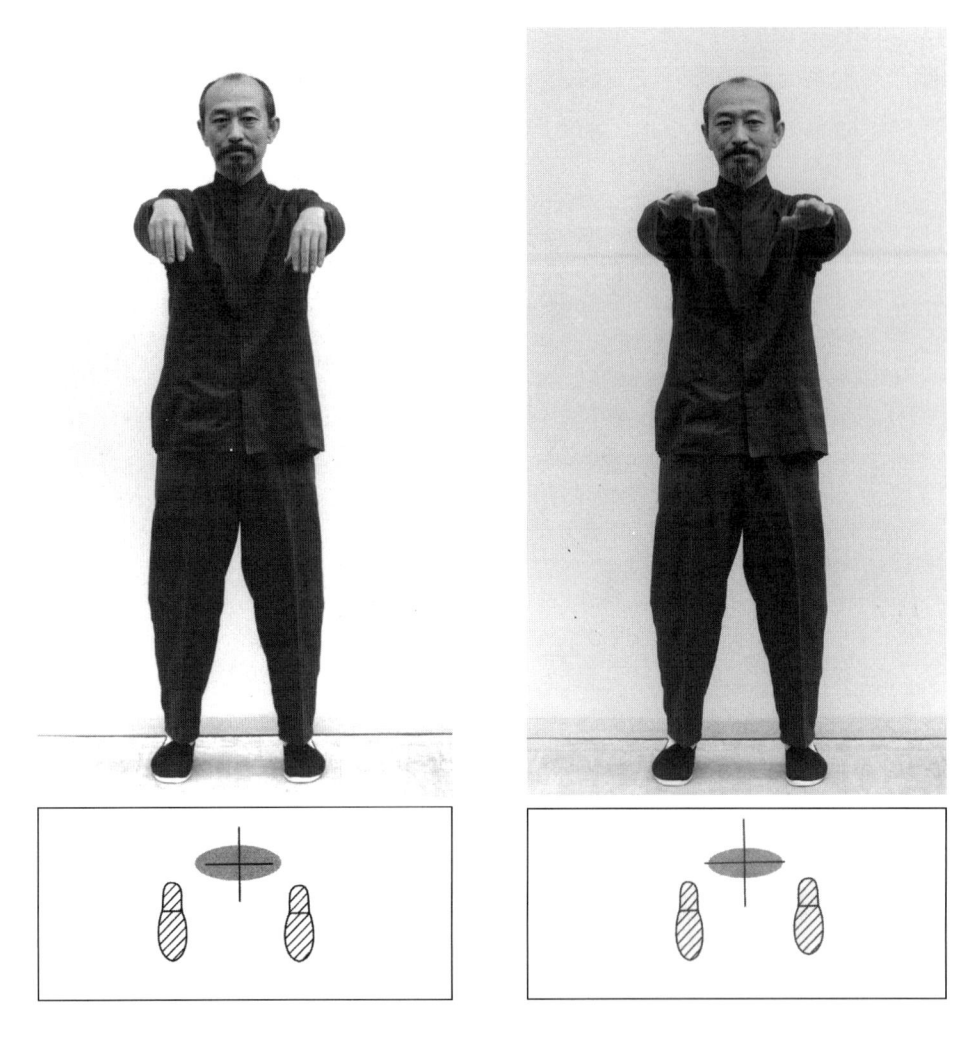

1. Raise the arms, relaxed, to shoulder height. At the same time, let the hands hang freely.

2. Through a release in the elbows that is almost indiscernible, raise the hands.

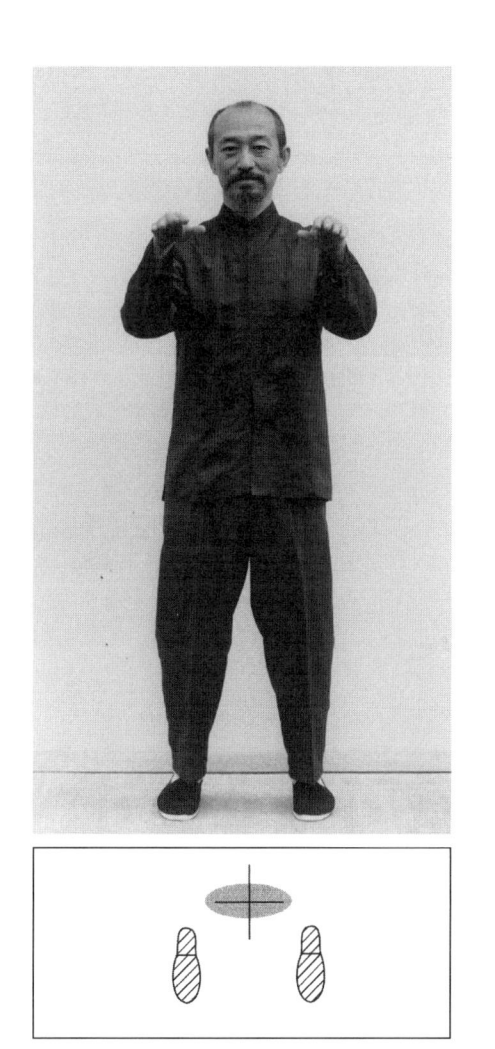

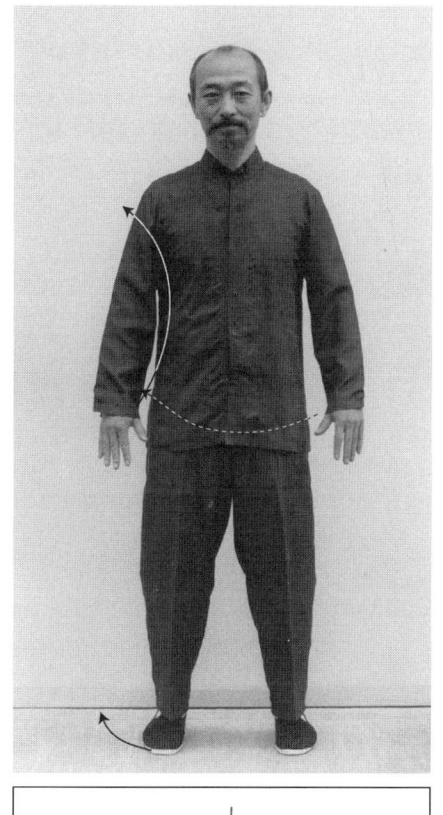

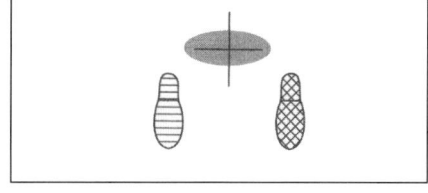

3. By bending the arms (release the elbows) pull the hands at shoulder level to the body.

Not shown: Lift the hands by further releasing the elbows.

4. Lower the arms, and at the same time lower the hands in a vertical line in front of the body. Conclude by somewhat bending both hands (standing hand). Simultaneously shift up to 70 percent of the weight onto the left foot.

3. Grasp the Sparrow's Tail—Ward-Off, Left

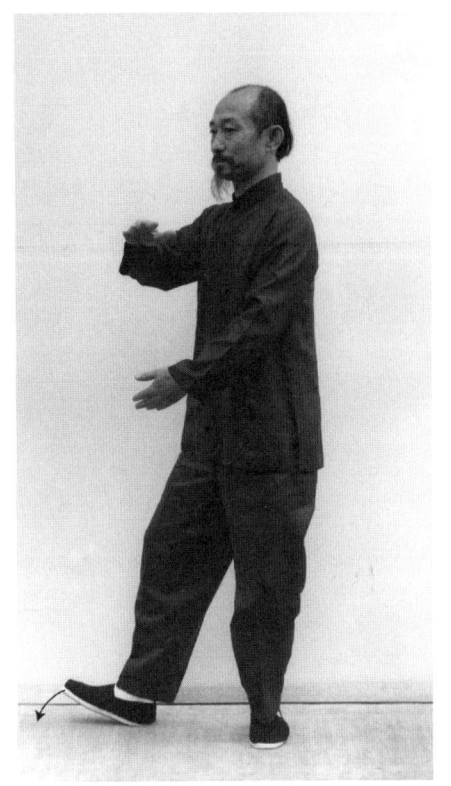

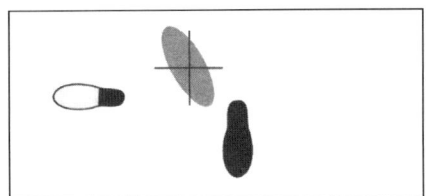

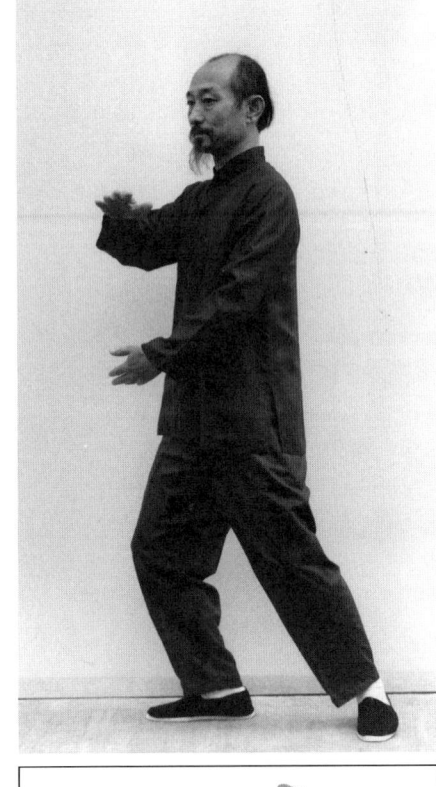

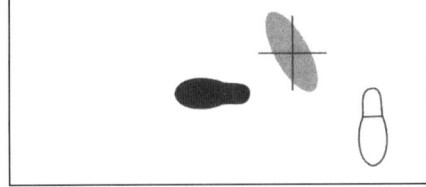

1. Turn the torso and right leg on the heel to the right until the front of the torso is facing NEE and the toes face E. At the same time, shift 90 percent of your weight onto the left foot and bend the knee. The arms follow the movement of the torso. Right arm: release in the elbow when lifting the arm. The lower arm and hand depict a half-circle in front of the body. Left arm: bring the arm in front of the body until the hand is in front of the central axis, turning the palm of the hand upward.

2. Shift up to 90 percent of the weight onto the right foot. At the same time, sink the foot and bend the knee. The position of the arms shouldn't change.

Note: The knee shouldn't go beyond the tip of the toes (the principle of the unity of the body in movement). Release in the right groin fold.

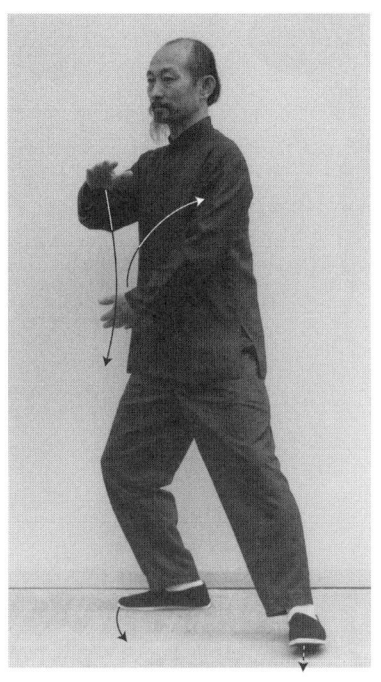

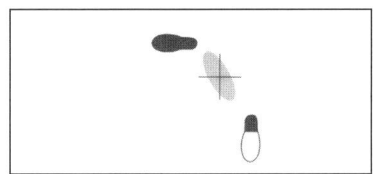

3. Place the left leg, heel first, straight forward (N).

Note: It is understood that in this and every other step your weight must first shift completely onto the foot that already carries 90 percent of the weight. While doing this, bend the knee further and continue to release in the groin fold.

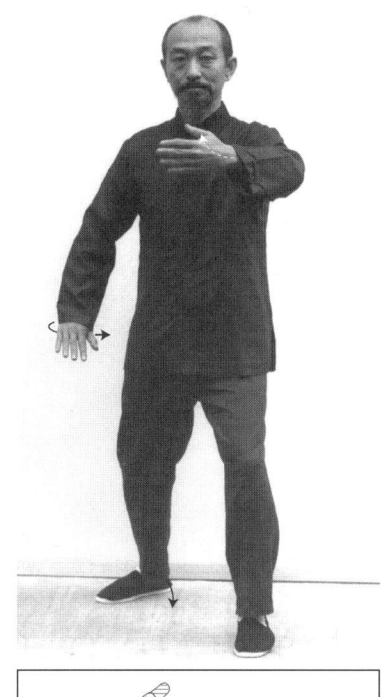

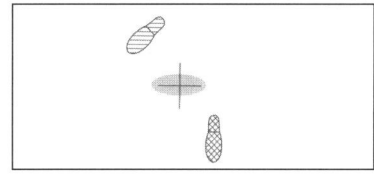

4. Turn the torso and right leg on the heel to the left until the front of the torso faces N and the tip of the toes face NE (Millstone Principle, Bow Step). At the same time, shift up to 70 percent of the weight onto the left foot, sink the foot, and bend the knee. The arms follow the movement of the torso: Lift the left arm, slightly rounded, until the hand is at the height of the breastbone, the palm faces the body. Lower the right arm. Toward the end of the movement, somewhat bend the hand (standing hand).

The left foot is in front and carries 70 percent of the weight; the right foot is in back with 30 percent.

You are in the position "Ward-Off, Left."

4. Grasp the Sparrow's Tail—Ward-Off, Right

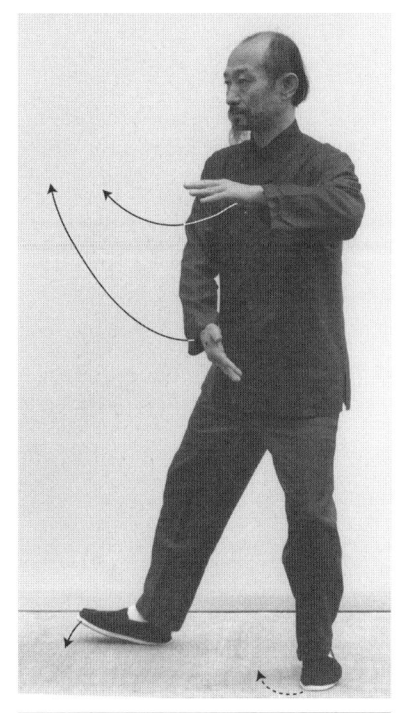

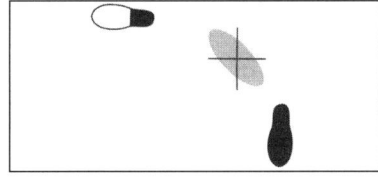

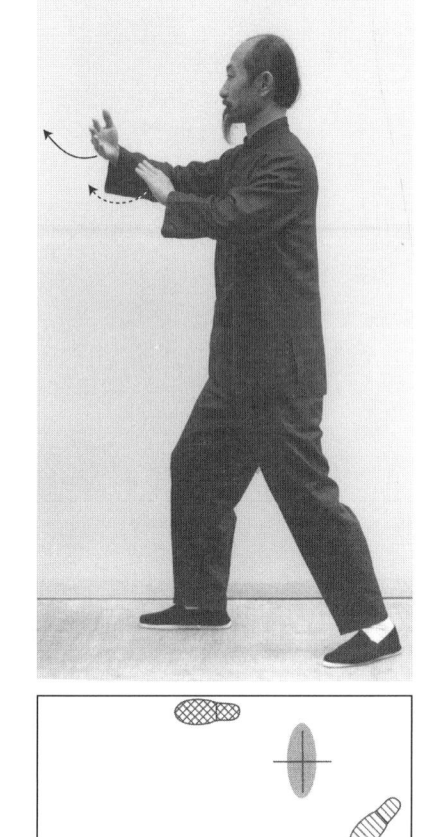

1. a) Turn the torso to the right until the front side faces NE. Simultaneously, shift up to 90 percent of the weight onto the left foot. The right leg follows the movement of the torso with lifted heel until the toes point E. Along with the shift of weight, turn the left hand until the palm faces downward and move the right arm in front of the body until the hand is in front of the central axis with the palm facing upward. You face NE.

b) Place the right leg, heel first, half a foot length in front (E). The weight remains on the left foot. The position of the arms stays the same. You face E.

2. Turn the torso and the left leg on the heel to the right until the front side of the torso faces E and the toes point NE (Millstone Principle, Bow Step). While doing this, shift up to 70 percent of the weight onto the right foot, sink the foot, and bend the knee. Simultaneously with the torso turn, raise the right arm slightly rounded. The left arm follows the movement of the torso. Toward the end of the movement, bring both arms somewhat forward and up, and bend the left hand slightly (standing hand).

70 percent of the weight rests on the front right foot, 30 percent on the back left foot.

You are in the position "Ward-Off, Right."

5. Grasp the Sparrow's Tail—Rollback

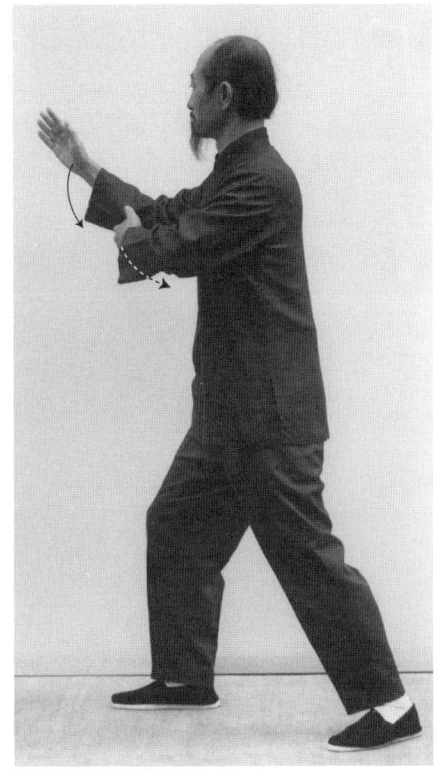

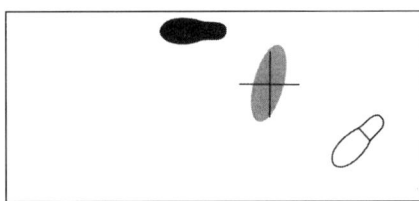

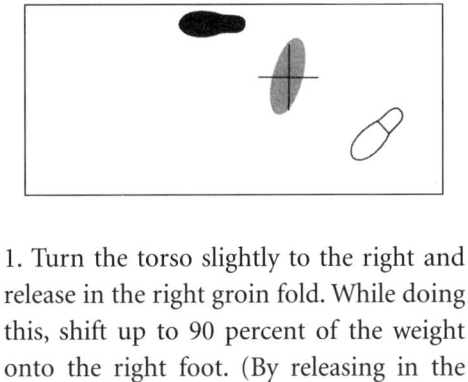

1. Turn the torso slightly to the right and release in the right groin fold. While doing this, shift up to 90 percent of the weight onto the right foot. (By releasing in the groin area, the torso turn occurs by itself, so to speak!)

The arms follow the movement of the torso. Right arm: the lower arm and hand turn counterclockwise as one unit from the elbow. Left arm: the lower arm and hand turn counterclockwise as one unit. The left hand approaches the right elbow.

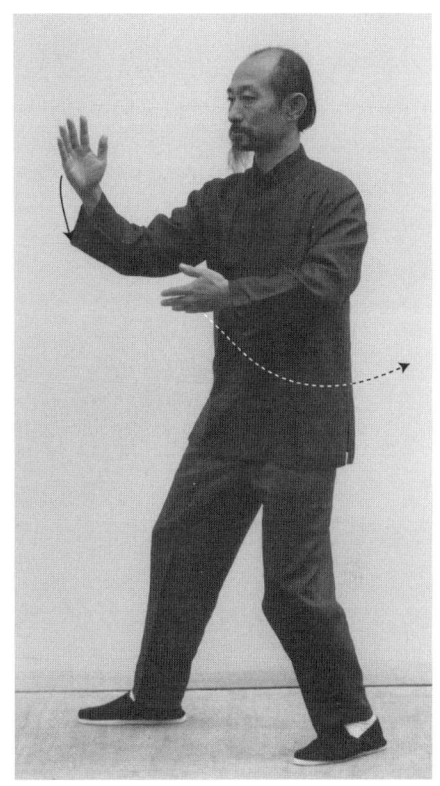

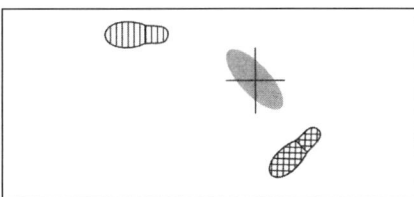

2. Turn the torso to the left until the front side faces NE. At the same time, shift up to 70 percent of the weight onto the left foot. The arms follow the movement of the torso. Release somewhat in both elbows.

70 percent of the weight rests on the back left foot and 30 percent on the front right foot.

You are in the position "Rollback."

Note: The turning of the torso to the left begins at the same time as the weight shift (Millstone Principle).

6. Grasp the Sparrow's Tail—Press

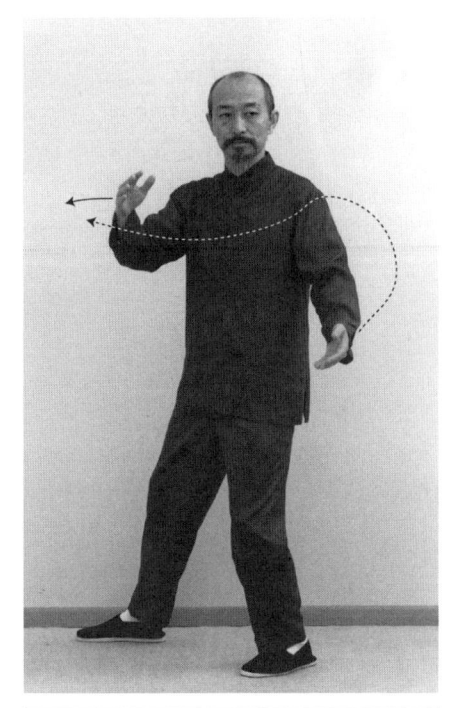

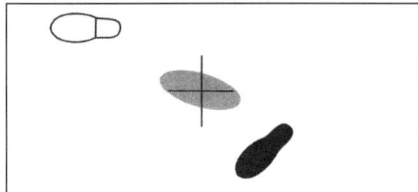

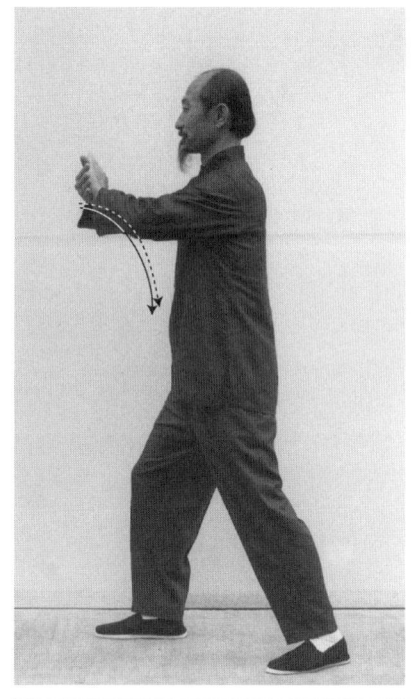

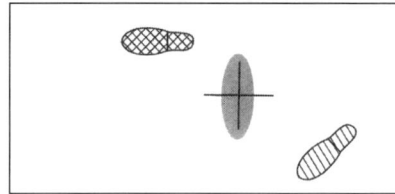

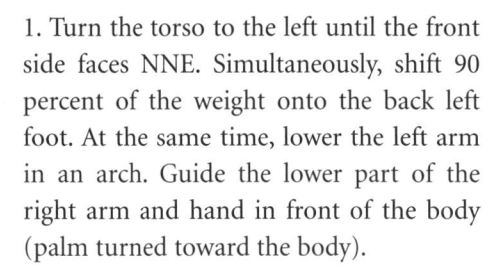

1. Turn the torso to the left until the front side faces NNE. Simultaneously, shift 90 percent of the weight onto the back left foot. At the same time, lower the left arm in an arch. Guide the lower part of the right arm and hand in front of the body (palm turned toward the body).

2. Turn the torso to the right until the front side faces E. At the same time, shift up to 70 percent of your weight onto the front right foot. The arms follow the movement of the torso. The position of the right arm remains the same. The left arm follows an upward arch in front of the body and, with a slight sinking, approaches the right hand. Toward the end of the movement, bring both arms slightly forward and up, thereby placing the left hand on the right inner wrist.

70 percent of the weight rests on the front right foot and 30 percent on the back left foot.

You are in the position "Press."

7. Grasp the Sparrow's Tail—Push

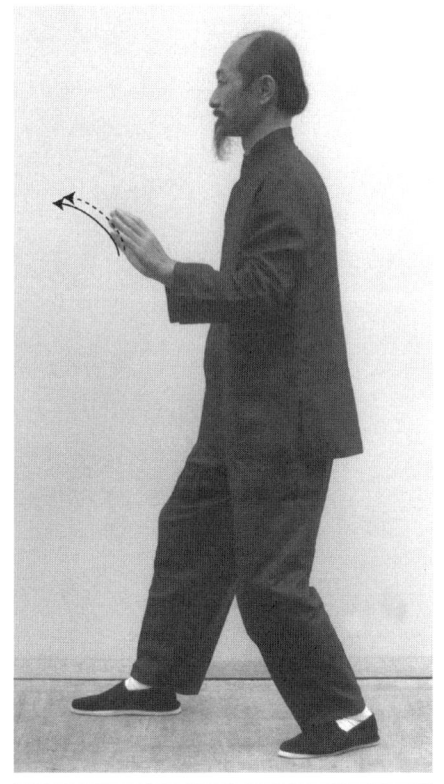

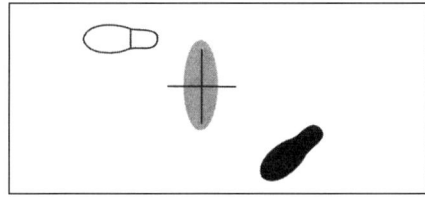

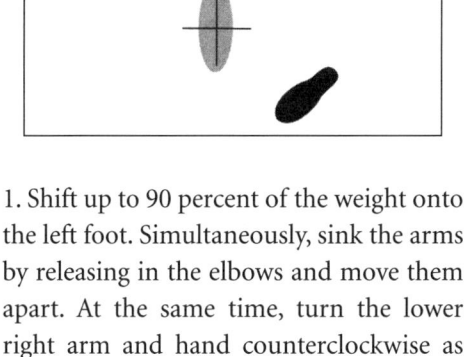

1. Shift up to 90 percent of the weight onto the left foot. Simultaneously, sink the arms by releasing in the elbows and move them apart. At the same time, turn the lower right arm and hand counterclockwise as one unit.

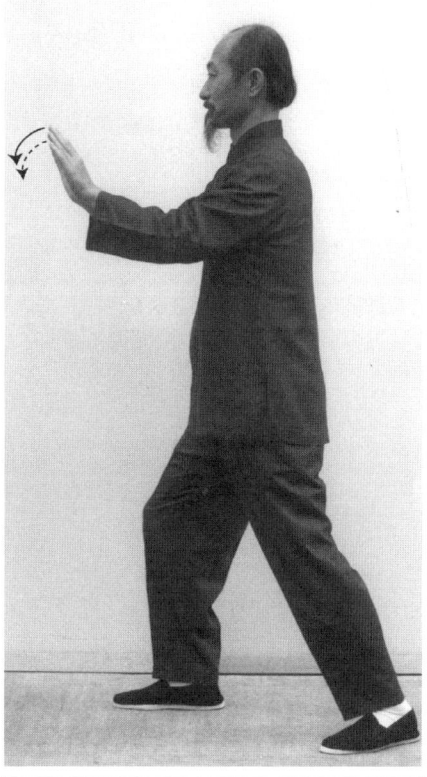

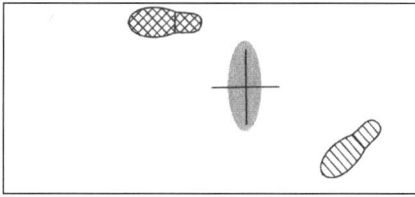

2. Shift up to 70 percent of the weight onto the right foot, and bend the knee. Bring the arms somewhat forward and up to push.

70 percent of the weight rests on the front right foot and 30 percent on the back left foot.

You are in the position "Push."*

---

* Depending on the situation, practitioners can use either the crossing energy path or the direct energy path in pushing.

8. Single Whip

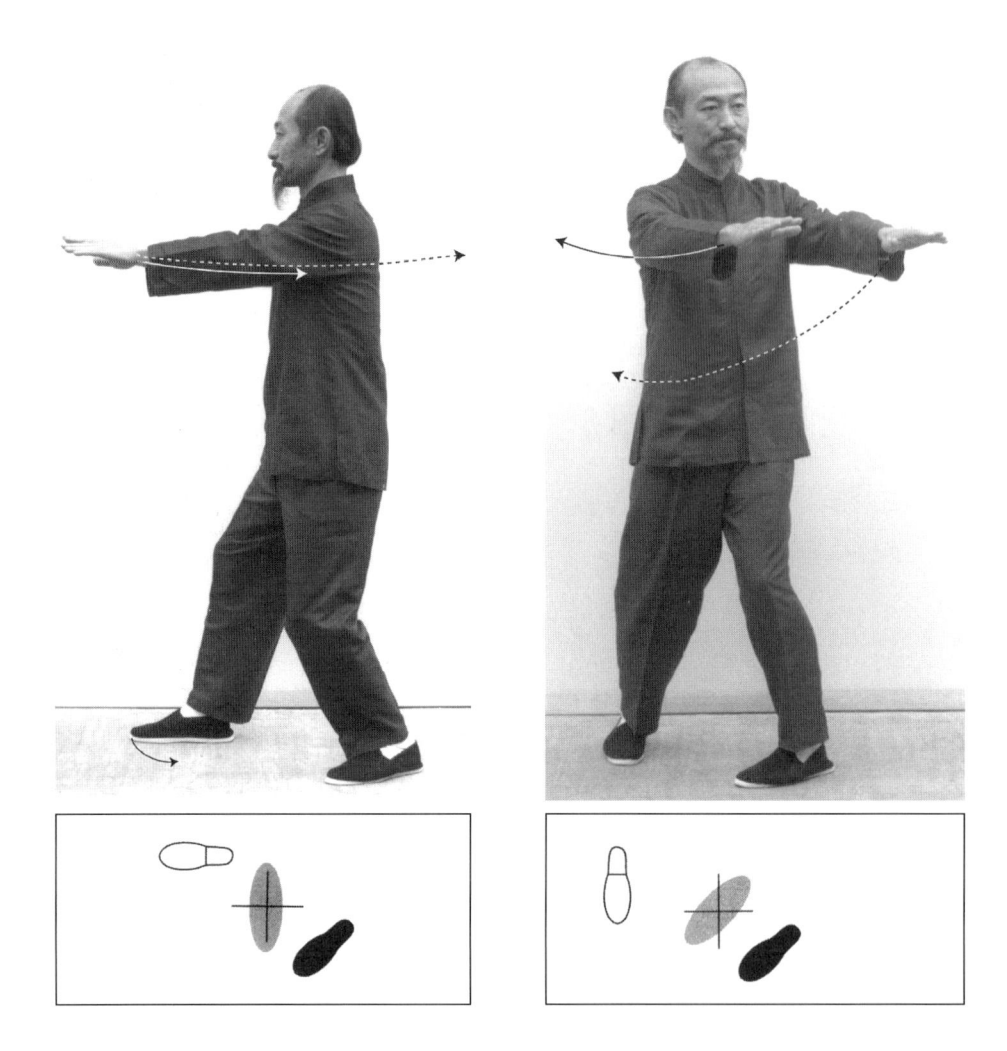

1. Shift up to 90 percent of the weight onto the left foot. The hands remain forward. (In this way, the arms stretch by themselves with the shifting backward). The palms of the hands face downward now.

2. Turn the torso and the right leg on the heel to the left until the front side faces NW and the toes face N. The arms follow the turning of the torso in their parallel position until the fingertips point NW.

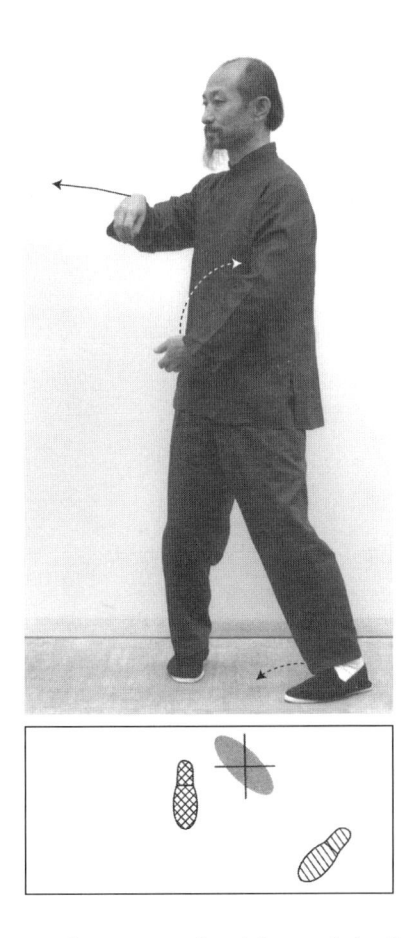

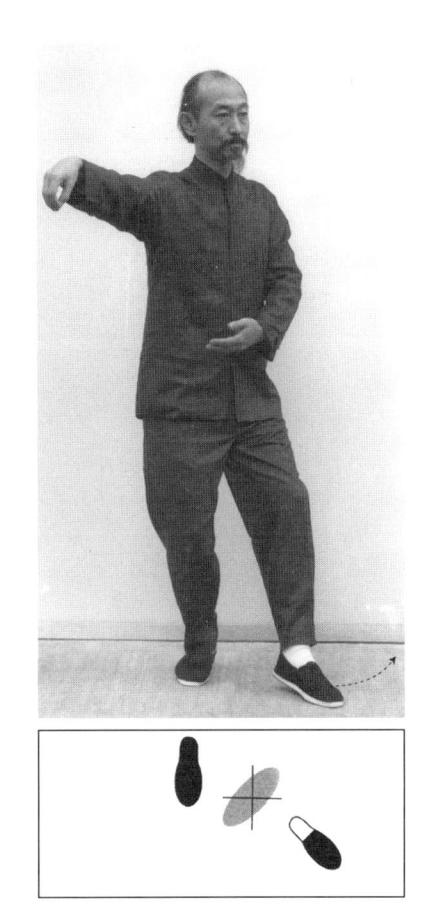

3. Turn the torso to the right until the front side faces NE. At the same time, shift up to 70 percent of the weight onto the right foot. The arms follow the movement of the torso. Left arm: lower the arm and bring it in front of the body until the left hand is in front of the right hip. (The palm of the hand faces upward.) Right arm: leaving the arm at the same height, bend it until it approaches the body (Elbow Strike). Lower the hand and close the fingertips into the Bird's Head (Hook Hand). The right and left hands are in a vertical line.

Note: The torso turn to the right begins at the same time as the weight shift (Millstone Principle).

4. Turn the torso to the left until the front side faces NW. At the same time, shift up to 90 percent of the weight onto the right foot.

The left leg follows the movement of the torso with a raised heel until the toes point NW. Simultaneously, lift the left arm slightly in front of the body (Ward-Off). The right arm follows the torso turn and stretches slightly upward to the NE. The position of the hand remains the same.

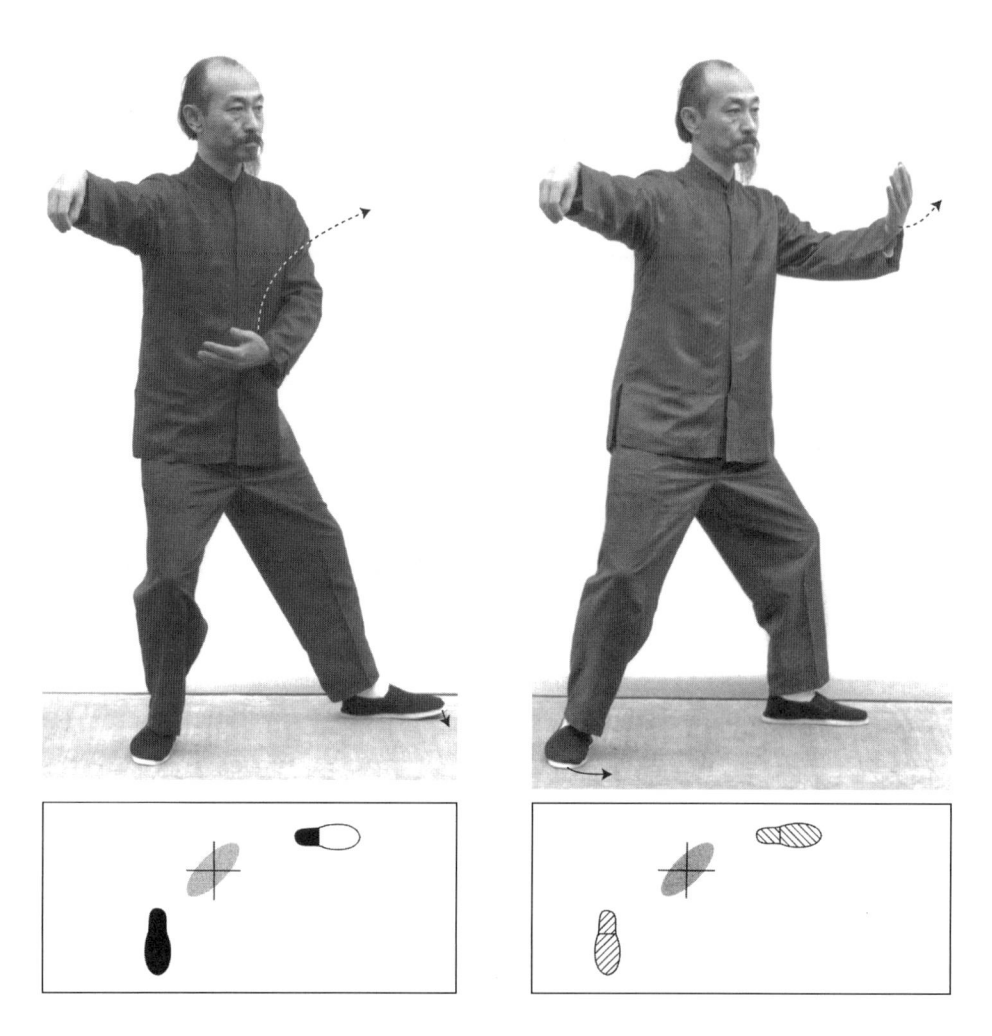

5. Place the left leg with the heel to the SW following an arch.

6. Turn the torso slightly left (Millstone Principle). While doing this, shift up to 50 percent of the weight onto the left foot. Sink the foot and bend the knee. The left arm follows the movement of the torso in a large upward-directed arch. When lifting the arm, the palm of the hand remains turned toward the body. The position of the right arm stays as it is.

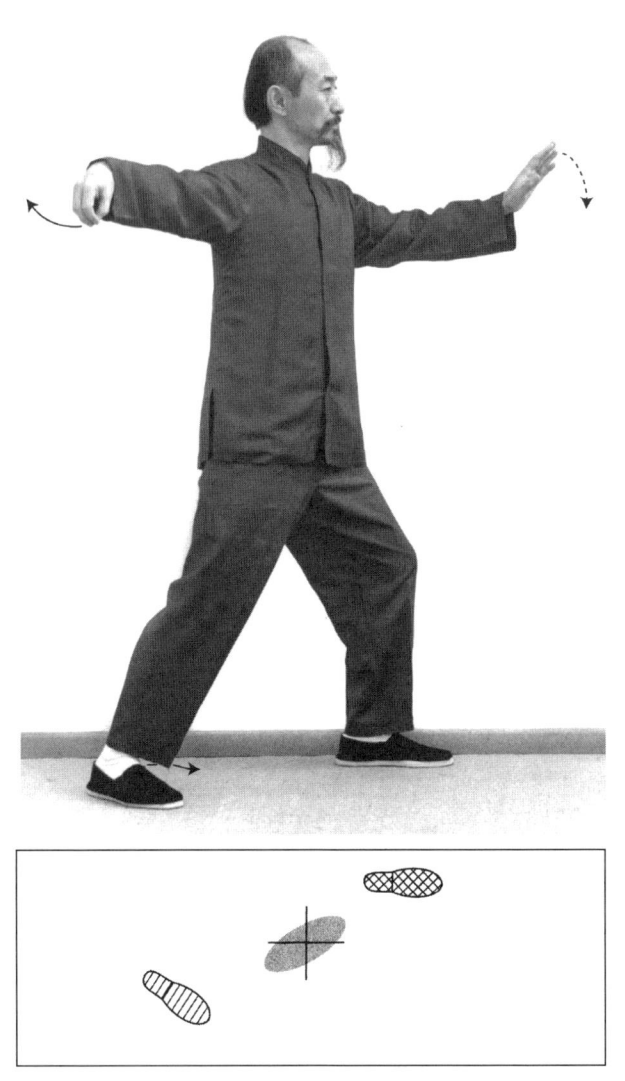

7. Turn the torso and right leg on the heel to the left until the front side of the torso faces NWW and the toes point NW (Millstone Principle, Bow Step). At the same time, shift up to 70 percent of your weight onto the left foot and bend the knee. Near the end of the movement, turn the left lower arm and hand forward, bending the hand slightly (standing hand), and indicate a push with it. Toward the end of the movement, slightly lift the right arm (bird's head).

70 percent of the weight rests on the front left foot and 30 percent on the back right foot. The front side of the torso faces NWW.

You are in the position "Single Whip."

9. Lift Hands

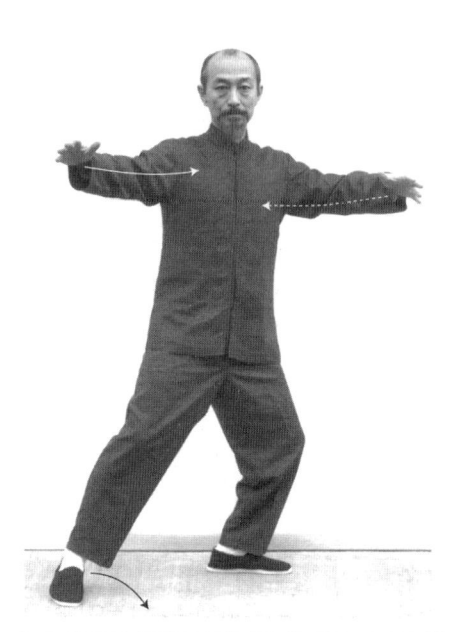

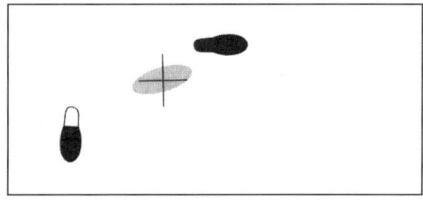

1. Turn the torso to the right until the front side faces NNW. Shift up to 90 percent of the weight onto the left foot. The right leg follows the movement of the torso with a raised heel until the toes point N.

Bring the arms slightly in by releasing in the elbows. At the same time, raise the right hand and open the "bird's head" by opening and separating the fingers.

You face N.

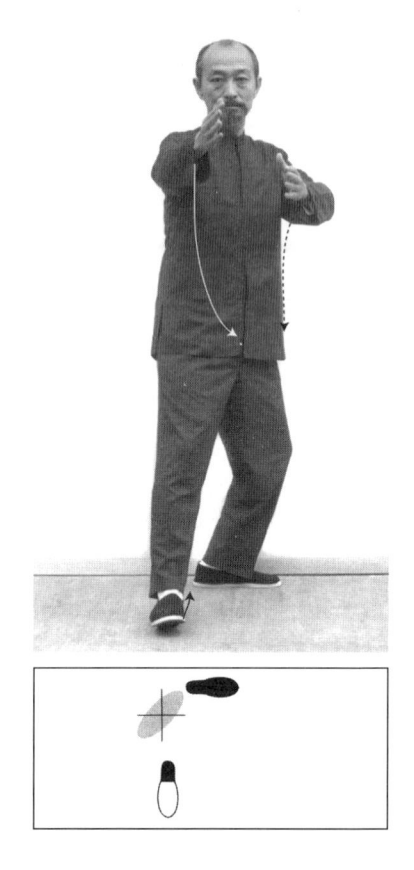

2. The weight remains on the left foot. Turn the torso slightly left until the front side faces NW. At the same time, the right leg follows in a slight arch to the left and is placed down and forward on the heel (T-Step). The leg isn't stretched out!

Simultaneously, bring both arms closer together by releasing in the elbows. At the same time, bring the left hand up to the height of the right elbow. The palms face the elbows.

90 percent of the weight rests on the back left foot and 10 percent on the front right foot.

You are in the position "Lift Hands."*

*The technique Split is used in the position "Lift Hands."

10. Shoulder Push (Lean Forward)

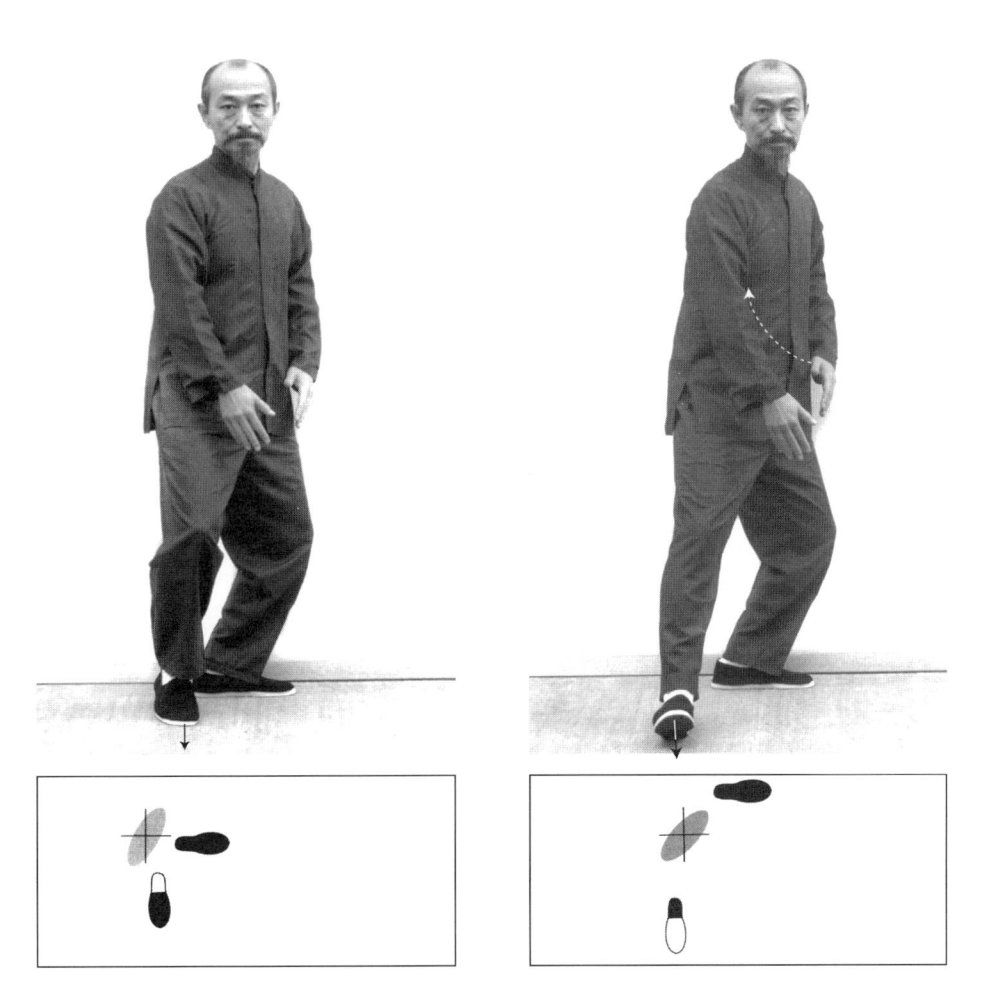

1. The weight remains on the left foot. Turn the torso slightly to the left until the front side faces NNW. At the same time, raise the right leg somewhat, pull it toward the body, and then lightly place the front part of the foot down. Simultaneously, lower the arms with the palms facing toward the body.

2. Turn the torso slightly to the right until the front side faces NW. While doing this, place the right leg directly forward on the heel (N).

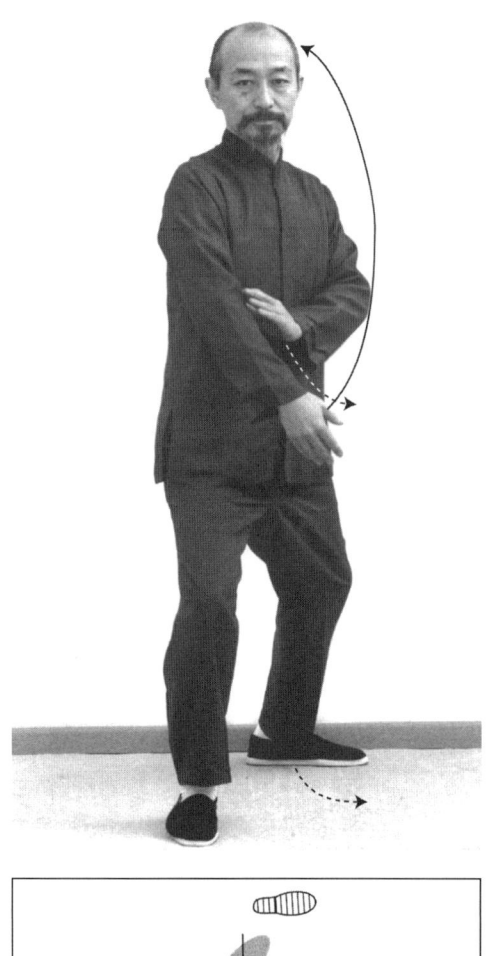

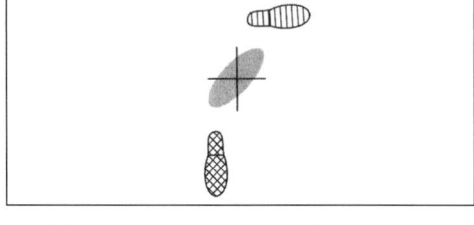

3. Shift up to 70 percent of the weight onto the right foot, sink the foot, and bend the knee. The right arm stays as it is, with the palm facing the body. Accompanying the shift of weight, lift the left lower arm and hand in front of the body. The left hand nears the crook of the right arm. Toward the end of the movement, slightly bend the left hand (standing hand).

The front side of the torso faces NW.

You face N.

70 percent of the weight rests on the front right foot and 30 percent on the back left foot.

You are in the position "Shoulder Push (Lean Forward)."

11. Stork Spreads Wings

1. Turn the torso to the left until the front side faces NNW. At the same time, shift the entire weight onto the right foot. Toward the end of the movement, the left leg follows an arch forward (W) and is placed down on the front part of the foot (Step of the Fishing Horse). Simultaneously, stretch the right leg somewhat. As the torso turns, lift the slightly rounded right arm. At the same time, turn the lower arm and hand as one unit (don't raise the shoulder!). Lower the left arm next to the side of the body. Toward the end of the movement, bend the hand slightly (standing hand).

90 percent of the weight rests on the back right foot and 10 percent on the front left foot. The front side of the torso faces NWW.

You face W.

You are in the position "Stork Spreads Wings."

Note: The torso turn must occur very slowly in order to coordinate with the large movement of the right arm.

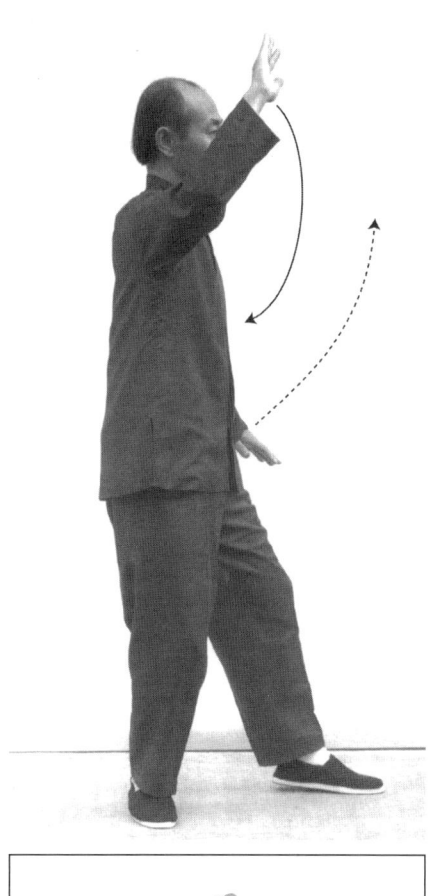

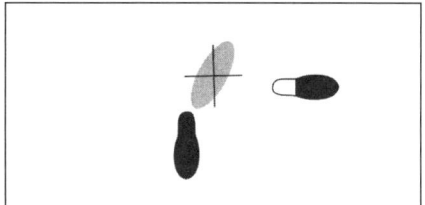

12. Brush Left Knee—Twist Step

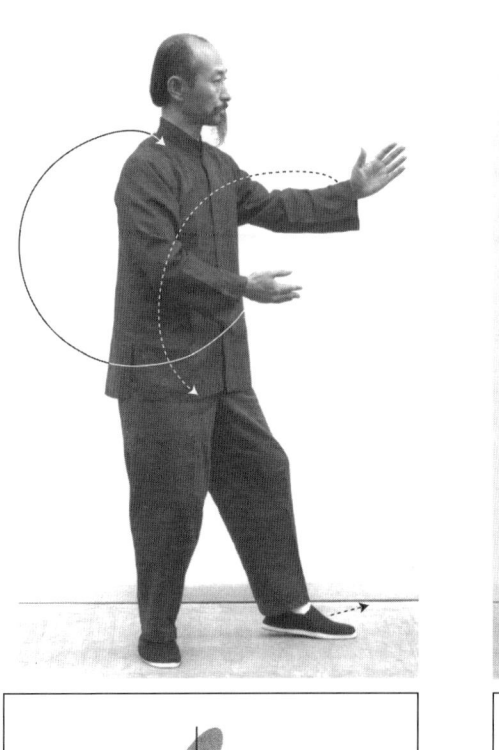

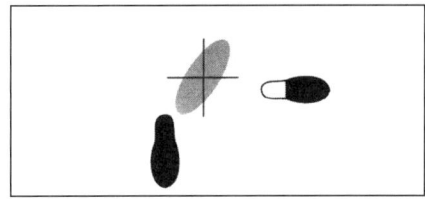

1. The weight remains on the right foot. Turn the torso slightly to the right. At the same time, bend the knee somewhat (release and sink). Simultaneously, begin the counter-rotating movement of the arms: lower the right arm (hand in front of the central axis) and lift the left arm at the side of the body.

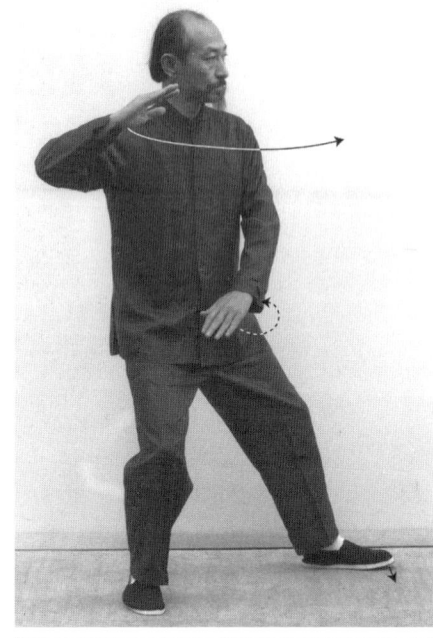

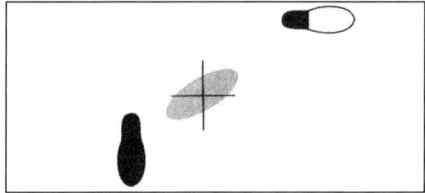

2. a) Turn the torso to the right until the front side faces NNW. Lift the right arm in an arch first to the height of the shoulder (the fingertips point NNE), and then guide the hand forward by bending the arm. Simultaneously, lower the left arm to the right in front of the body until the hand is in front of the right hip.

b) Place the left leg with the heel to the SW.

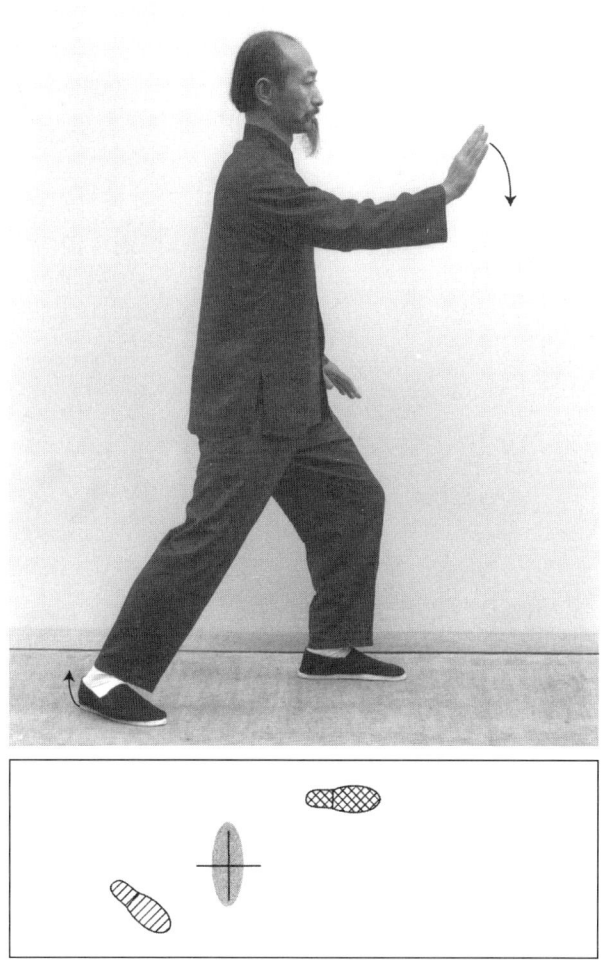

3. Turn the torso and the right leg on the heel to the left until the front side faces W and the toes point NW (Millstone Principle). At the same time, shift up to 70 percent of the weight onto the left foot, sink the foot, and bend the knee.

The arms follow the movement of the torso. Bring the right arm forward. Toward the end of the movement, bend the hand slightly (standing hand), and indicate a push. Guide the left arm to the left side of the body.

Bend the hand slightly (standing hand) to complete the movement.

70 percent of the weight rests on the front left foot and 30 percent on the back right foot.

You are in the position "Brush Left Knee—Twist Step."*

---

*This movement was originally performed much more deeply; the hand actually brushed the knee.

13. Play the Lute

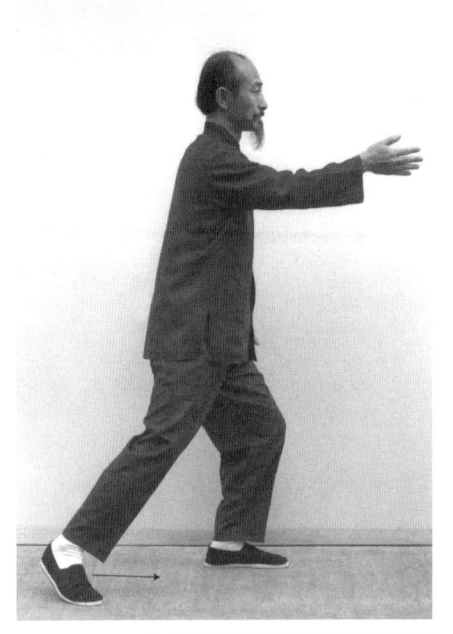

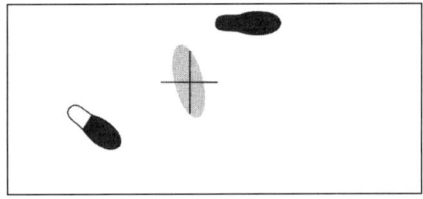

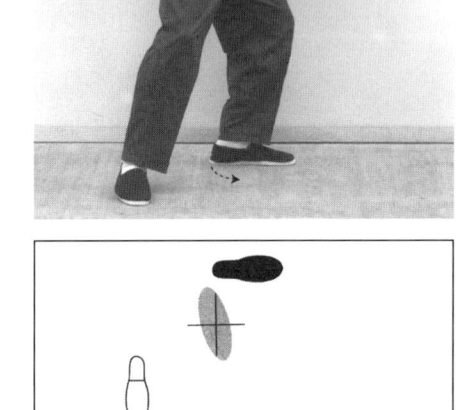

1. Turn the torso left until the front side faces SWW. At the same time, shift up to 90 percent of your weight onto the left foot and bend the knee (release in the groin fold).

Simultaneously, lower the right arm somewhat by releasing in the elbow, and turn the hand slightly clockwise. The position of the left arm remains the same. As your torso turns, slightly lift the heel of the right foot.

2. Place the right leg somewhat forward. Place the heel of the foot first, with the toes pointing N.

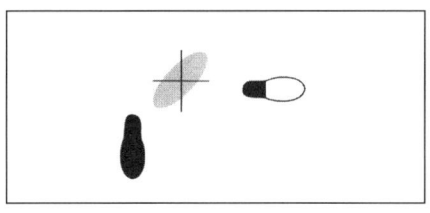

3. Turn the torso to the right until the front side faces NW. At the same time, shift up to 90 percent of your weight onto the right foot and bend the knee. Accompanying the torso turn, the left leg follows a small arch with the heel placed to the left. While doing this, lift the left arm forward and upward, turning the lower arm and hand slightly counterclockwise. Pull the right arm to the body by releasing in the elbow.

At the same time, the lower arm and hand turn somewhat counterclockwise. Finally, bend the right hand slightly (standing hand).

90 percent of the weight rests on the back right foot and 10 percent on the front left foot. The front side of the torso faces NW. You face W.

You are in the position "Play the Lute."

Repetition

Brush Left Knee—Twist Step (12)

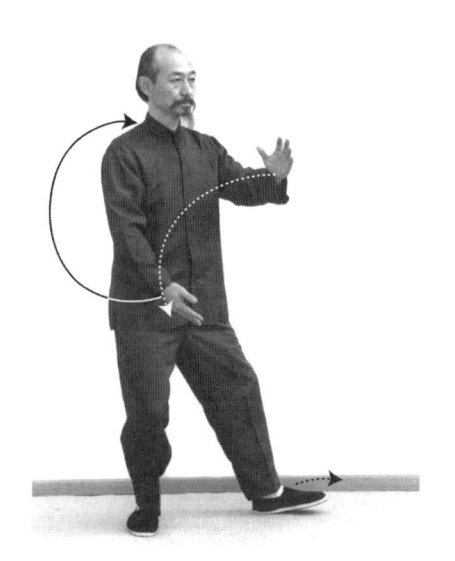

1. Bend the right knee somewhat (release, sink). At the same time, begin the torso turn to the right. The arms follow the movement of the torso (see position 12, photos 2–3).

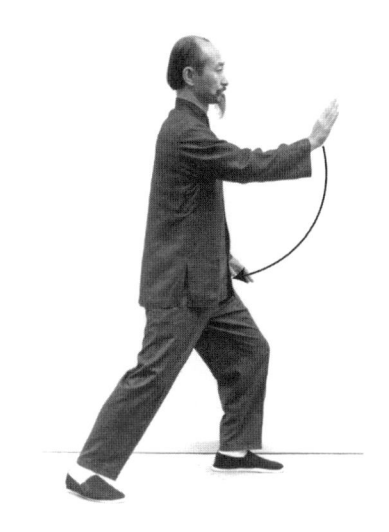

You are in the position "Brush Left Knee—Twist Step."

14. Step Forward, Deflect Downward, Parry, and Punch

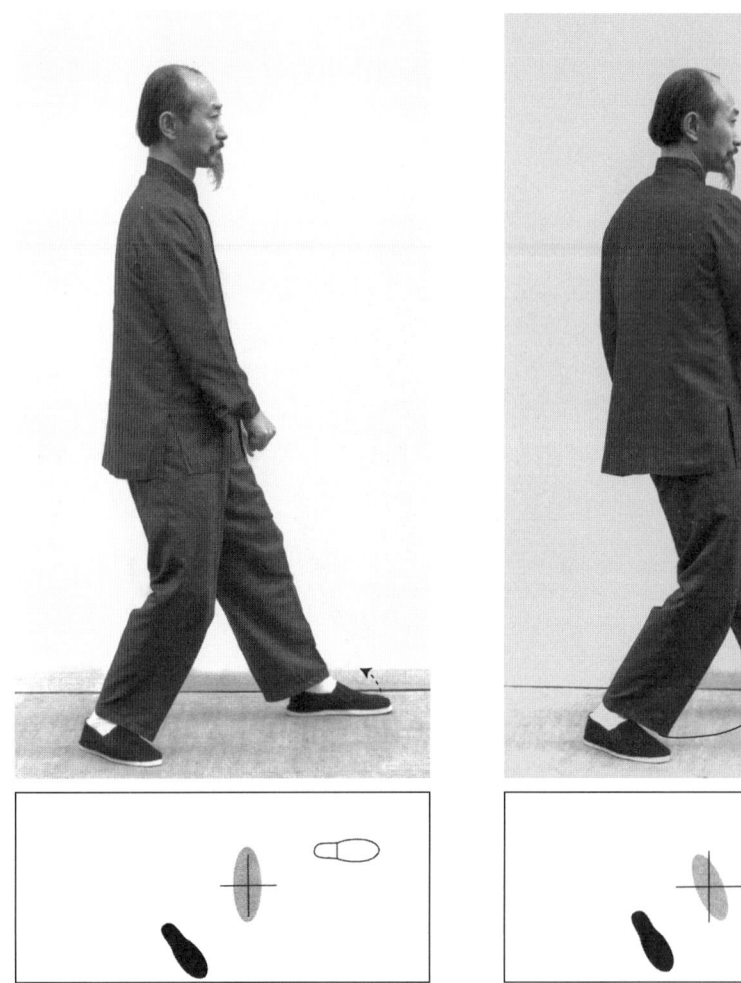

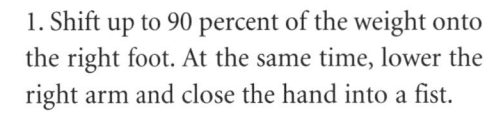

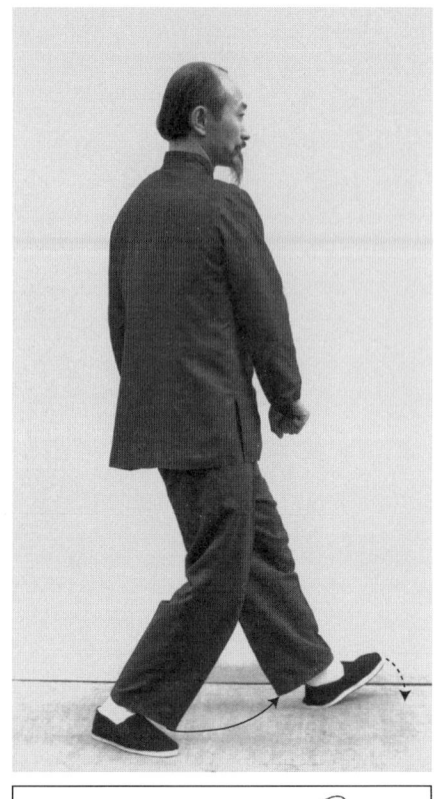

1. Shift up to 90 percent of the weight onto the right foot. At the same time, lower the right arm and close the hand into a fist.

2. Turn the torso and the left leg on the heel to the left until the front side of the torso faces SWW and the toes point SW. At the same time, turn the left hand somewhat counterclockwise.*

* In the application (self-defense), the movements shown in the photos 1 and 2 are carried out simultaneously.

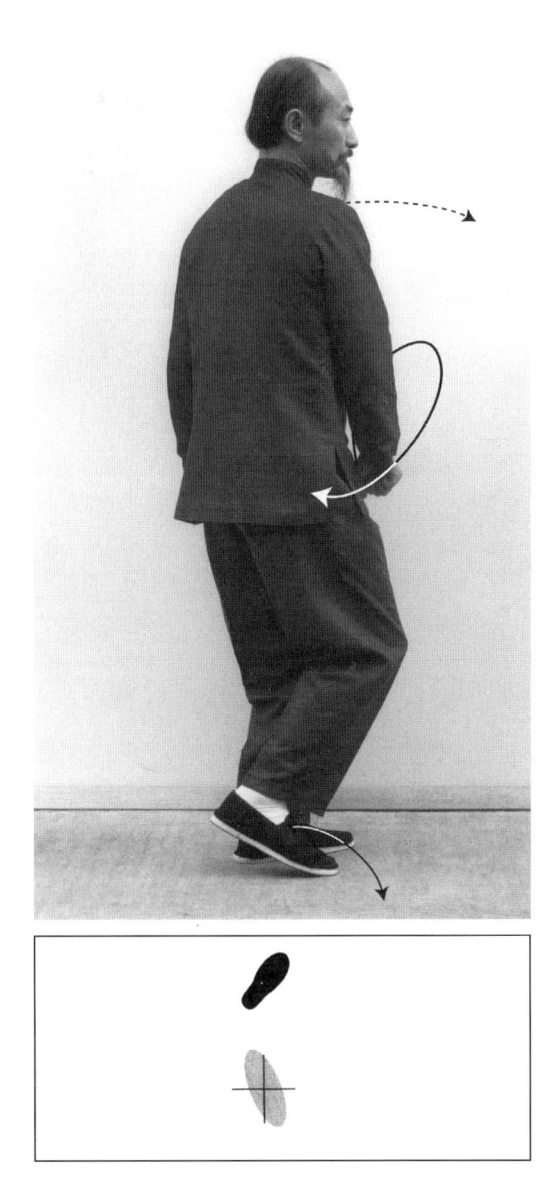

3. a) Shift the weight completely onto the left foot, sink the foot, and bend the knee.

b) Lift the right leg and pull it to the left. The position of the arms remains the same.

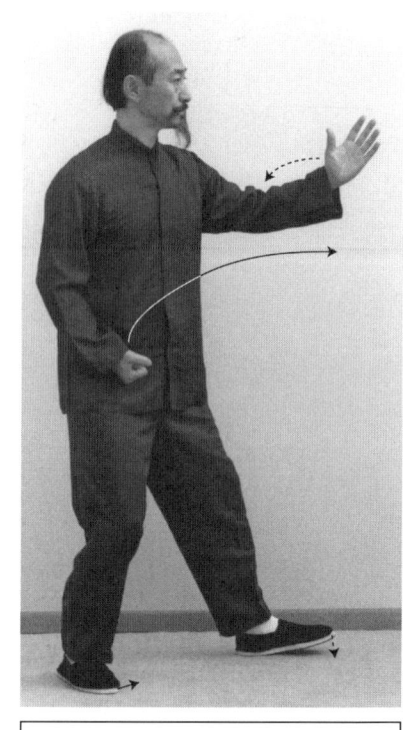

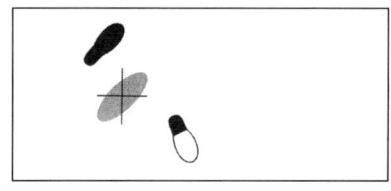

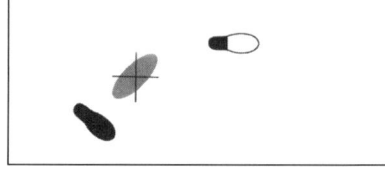

4. Standing on the left leg, turn the torso to the right until the front side faces NW. At the same time, place the right leg to the NW with the toes pointing NNW. The weight stays on the left foot. The arms follow the movement of the torso.

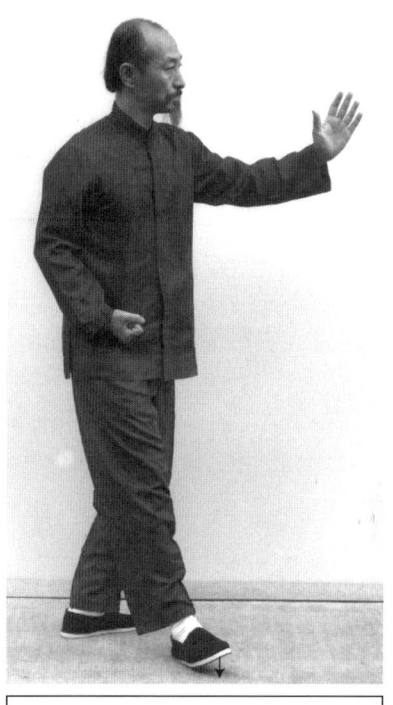

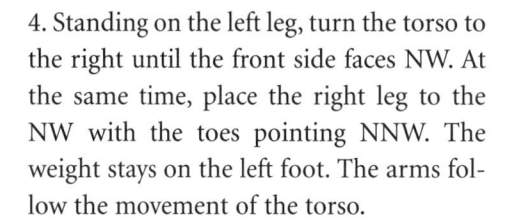

Both arms first follow an arch that guides them upward to the right (releasing in the elbows). Then bring the right arm to the right side of the body and pull the fist to the right hip. The back of the hand faces down.

Simultaneously, guide the left arm somewhat forward (W). The outer edges of the hands face W.

5. a) Shift up to 90 percent of the weight onto the right foot, sink the foot and bend the knee.

b) Place the left leg with the heel forward (W). The position of the arms stays the same.

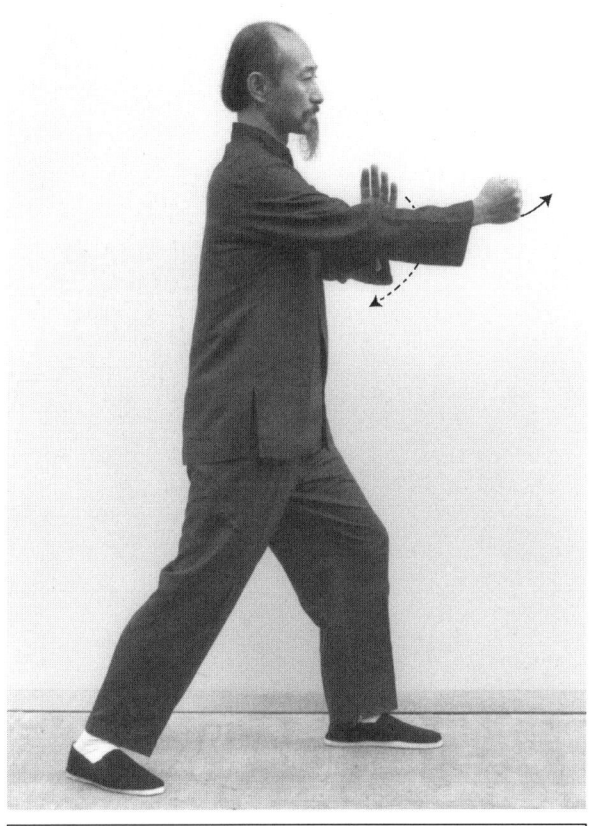

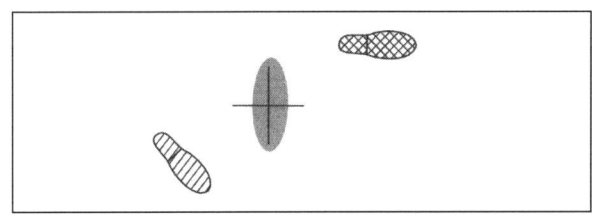

6. Turn the torso and the right leg on the heel to the left until the front side of the torso faces W and the toes point NW (Millstone Principle, Bow Step). At the same time, shift up to 70 percent of the weight onto the left foot.

Simultaneously, bring the fist forward from the hip in a somewhat inward (W) directed arch.*

In this movement, turn the lower arm and fist counterclockwise as one unit.

By releasing the elbow of the left arm, guide the left hand near to the body until the left hand is at the height of the crook of the elbow of the right arm.

70 percent of the weight rests on the front left foot and 30 percent on the back right foot.

You are in the position "Step Forward, Deflect Downward, Parry, and Punch."

* See page 84.

15. Withdraw and Push

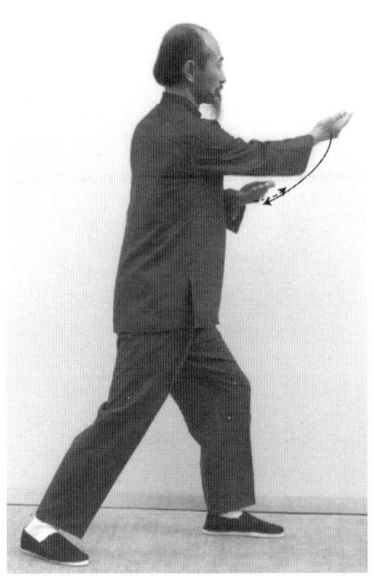

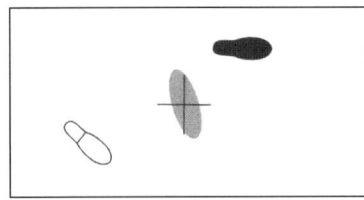

1. Turn the torso to the left until the front side faces SWW. At the same time, shift up to 90 percent of the weight onto the left foot. Simultaneously, stretch somewhat the right arm to the SWW, opening the fist and turning the palm of the hand upward. The left lower arm and hand sink in front of the body in a counterclockwise arch until the left hand is under the right elbow. The palm of the hand faces upward.

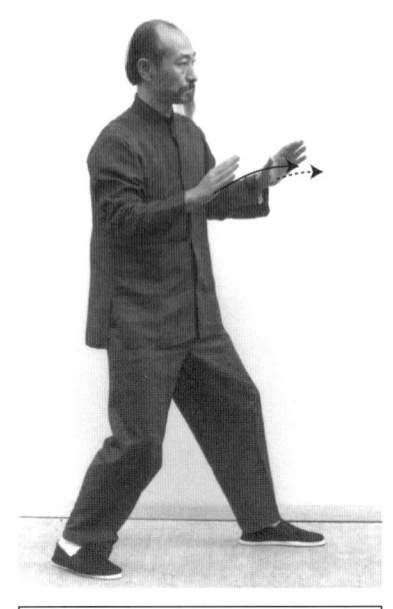

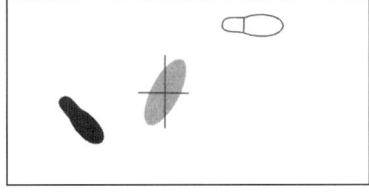

2. Turn the torso to the right until the front side faces NWW (Millstone Principle, Bow Step). While doing so, shift up to 90 percent of the weight onto the right foot. Right arm: (a) Pull the lower arm and hand over the palm of the left hand. (b) Bend the arm and, by releasing in the elbow, guide it to the right side of the body. At the same time, turn the lower arm and hand counterclockwise as one unit until the palm of the hand faces forward and downward.

Left arm: Guide the arm to the left side of the body by releasing in the elbow. At the same time, turn the lower arm and hand clockwise until the palm of the hand faces forward and downward.

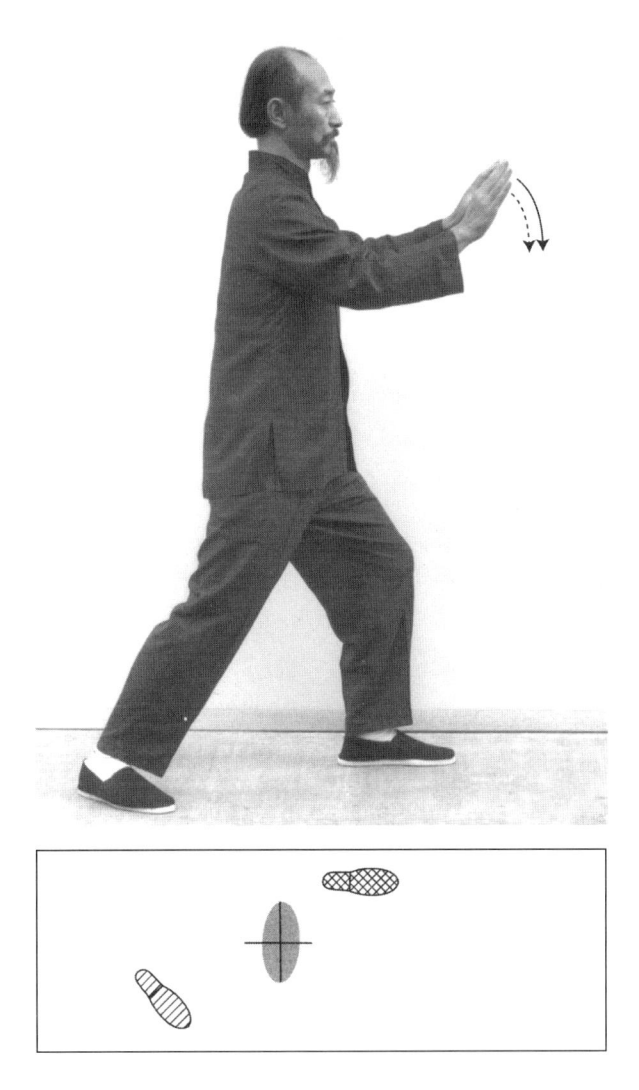

3. Turn the torso to the left until the front side faces W (Millstone Principle). At the same time, shift up to 70 percent of your weight onto the front left foot. Simultaneously, bring the arms to "push" somewhat forward and upward. 70 percent of the weight rests on the front left foot and 30 percent on the back right foot.

You are in the position "Withdraw and Push."

16. Cross Hands

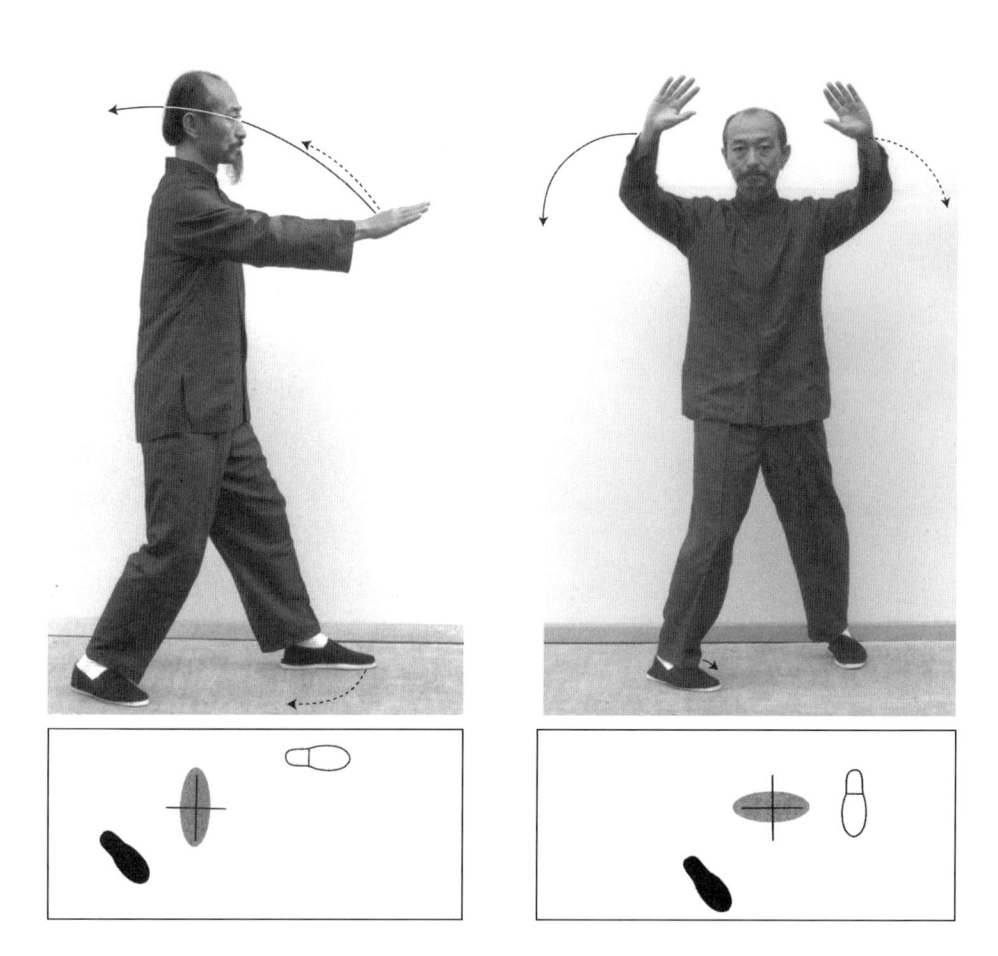

1. Shift up to 90 percent of the weight onto the back right foot. The hands remain forward. The arms seem to stretch by themselves. The palms of the hands face the floor.

2. Turn the torso to the right until the front side faces N. Simultaneously, turn the left foot on the heel until the toes point N. The weight remains on the right foot. The arms follow the movement of the torso. Raise both arms and move them apart from each other by placing the elbows outward. The palms of the hands face forward.

3. Shift up to 90 percent of the weight onto the left foot. While doing so, move the arms away from each other again and lower them to chest height.

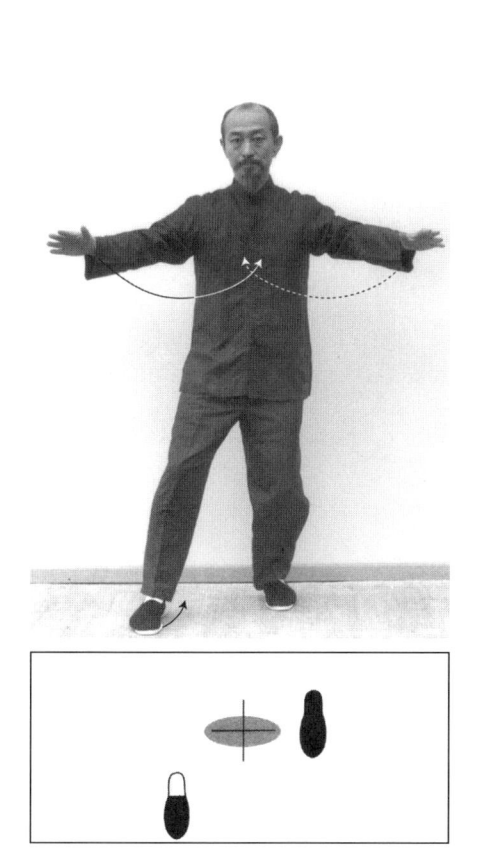

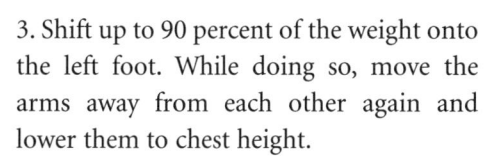

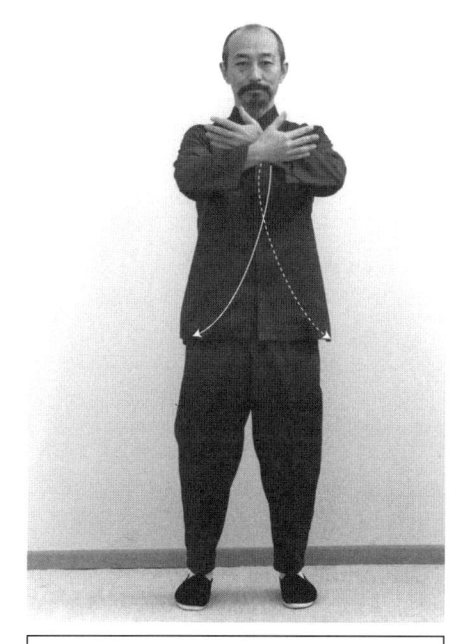

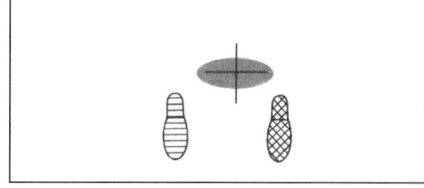

4. a) Place the right foot parallel to the left foot.

b) Shift up to 30 percent of the weight onto the right foot. At the same time, the arms come together in front of the body, following arches, until the wrists cross in front of the breastbone. The left hand is inside and both palms of the hands are turned toward the body.

70 percent of the weight rests on the left foot and 30 percent on the right foot.

You are in the position "Cross Hands."

Part 2

17. Embrace Tiger and Return to Mountain

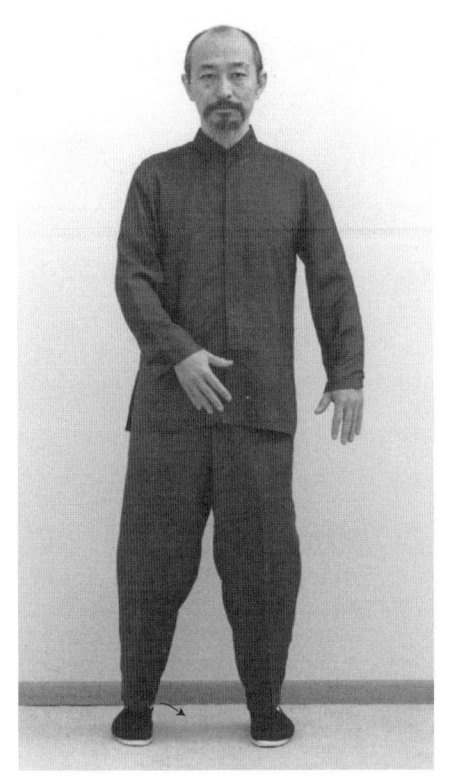

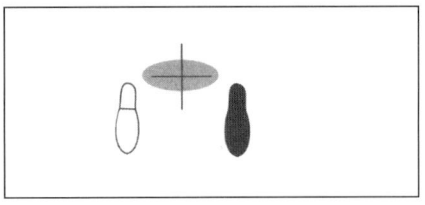

1. Shift up to 90 percent of the weight onto the left foot and bend the knee (release, sink). Simultaneously, lower both arms and move them apart from each other. The palms are turned toward the body.*

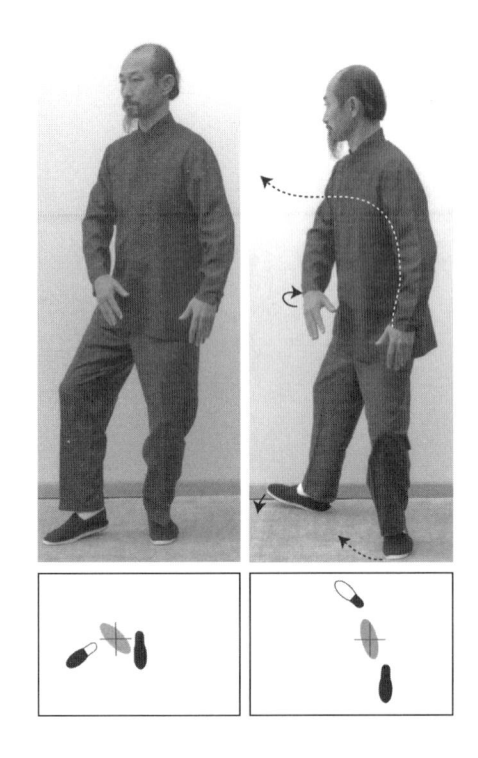

2. Turn the torso to the right until the front side faces NE. The right leg follows this movement with a raised heel until the toes point NE. The position of the arms remains the same.

3. Turn the torso to the right until the front side faces NEE. At the same time, place the right leg backward and to the right (SE) with the heel. Simultaneously, lift the left arm to the N (as in Brush Knee). The right arm follows the movement of the torso.

---

* In the first part of the short form, the positions only face N, E, or W. In the second and third parts of the short form, they also face NE, SE, SW, or NE. This is called "Corner Work"; the movement is directed diagonally to the corners.

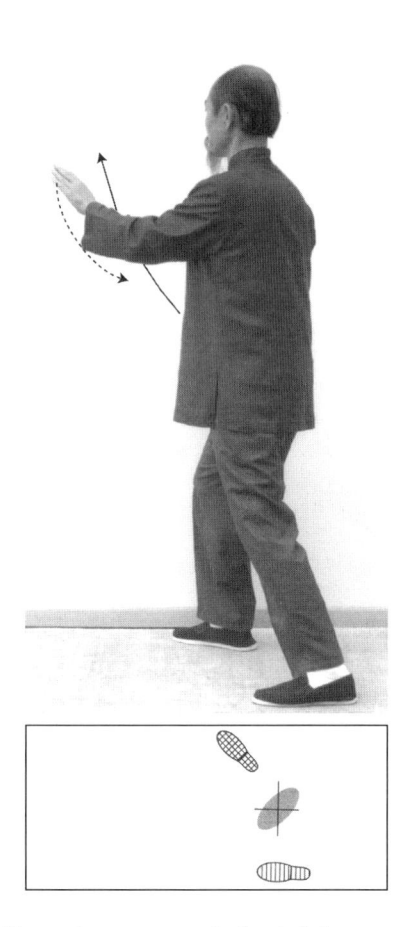

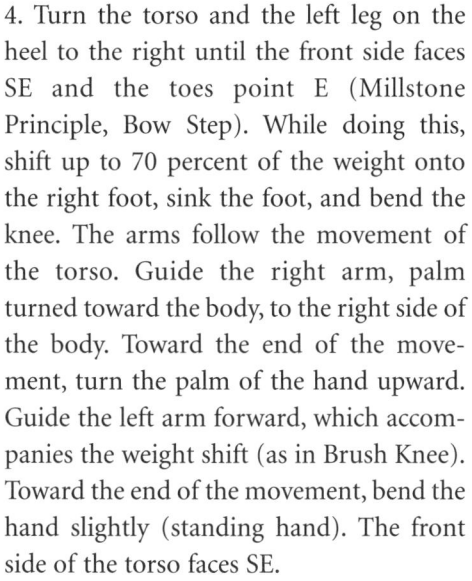

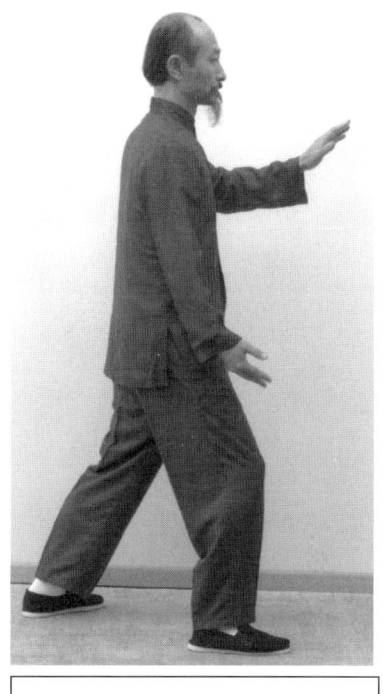

4. Turn the torso and the left leg on the heel to the right until the front side faces SE and the toes point E (Millstone Principle, Bow Step). While doing this, shift up to 70 percent of the weight onto the right foot, sink the foot, and bend the knee. The arms follow the movement of the torso. Guide the right arm, palm turned toward the body, to the right side of the body. Toward the end of the movement, turn the palm of the hand upward. Guide the left arm forward, which accompanies the weight shift (as in Brush Knee). Toward the end of the movement, bend the hand slightly (standing hand). The front side of the torso faces SE.

70 percent of the weight rests on the front right foot and 30 percent on the back left foot.

You are in the position "Embrace Tiger and Return to Mountain."*

*This position contains the technique Bend Backward.

Repetition

Rollback (5)

1. a) Turn the torso slightly to the left until the front side faces SEE (Millstone Principle). At the same time, shift up to 70 percent of the weight onto the left foot and bend the knee. Simultaneously, lift the right arm forward, lower the left arm, and guide the arms as in "Rollback" together.*

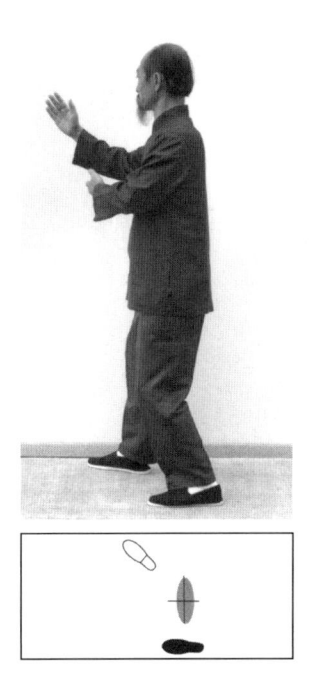

b) Turn the torso further to the left until the front side faces E. While doing so, shift up to 90 percent of the weight onto the left foot. The arms follow the movement of the torso. You repeat "Rollback."

90 percent of the weight rests on the back left foot and 10 percent on the front right foot.

You are in the position "Rollback."

* In the "Rollback" in the first part of the short form, an attack is yielded to with most of the weight on the front foot. In this case, most of the weight is on the back foot.

Press (6) facing SE
Push (7) facing SE
Single Whip (8) facing NW

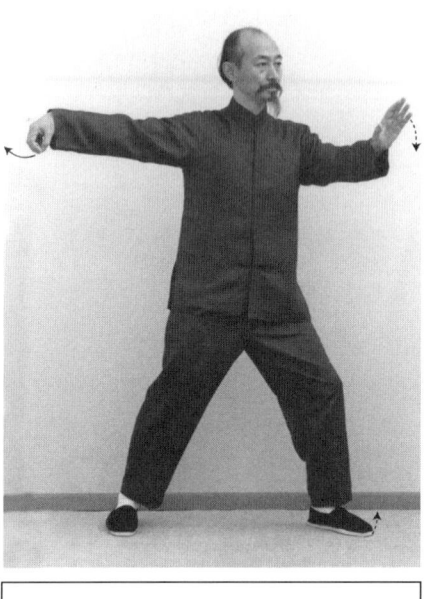

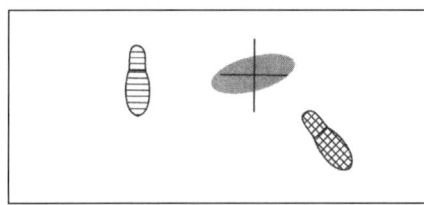

1. You are in the position "Single Whip," facing NW. The front side of the torso faces NNW.

18. Fist under Elbow

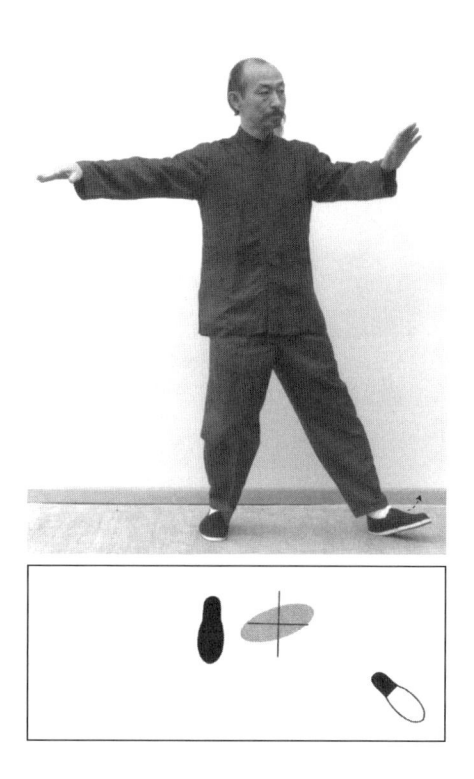

1. Shift up to 90 percent of the weight onto the back right foot and bend the right knee. At the same time, lift the front part of the left foot. Slightly release both elbows. Lower the lower arm and hand of the left arm. Lift the right hand and open the "Bird's Head" by moving the fingers apart.

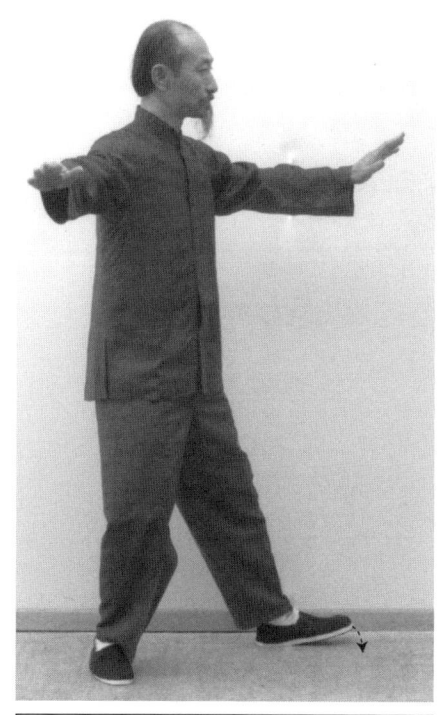

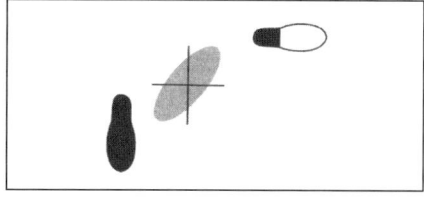

2. Turn the torso somewhat to the left until the front side faces NW. At the same time, place the left leg to the left with the heel, the toes pointing W. The arms follow the movement of the torso in the same positions as before.

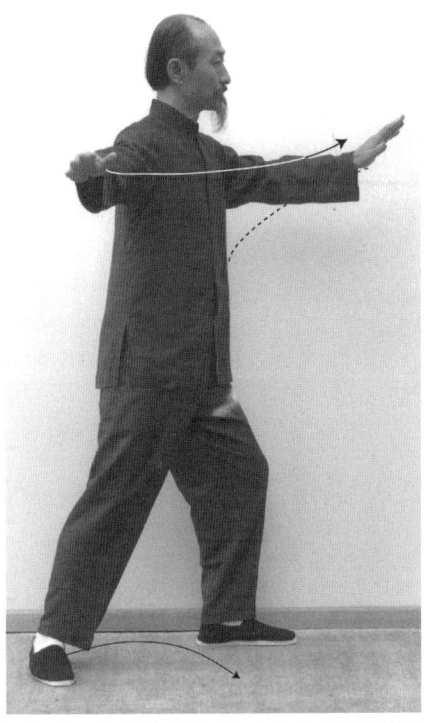

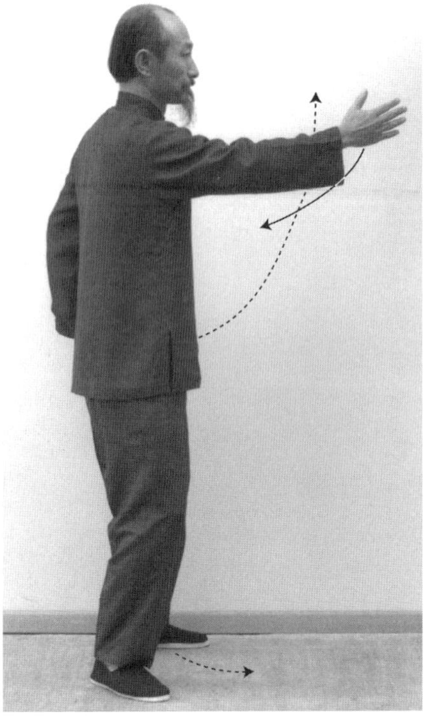

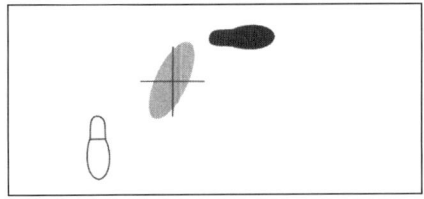

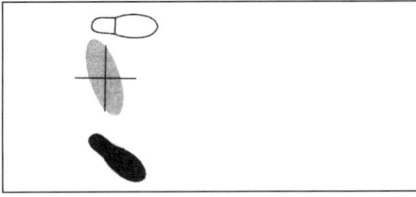

3. a) Turn the torso to the left until the front side faces NWW. At the same time, shift up to 90 percent of the weight onto the left foot and bend the knee. The arms follow the movement of the torso in the same positions as before.

b) Place the right leg to the NW, heel first. The toes point NW.

4. Turn the torso left until the front side faces SWW. At the same time, shift up to 90 percent of the weight onto the right foot. The right arm follows the movement of the torso until the fingertips point W. At the same time, turn the lower arm and hand slightly clockwise. The left arm follows the movement of the torso and then sinks extended out (hand to the hip level).

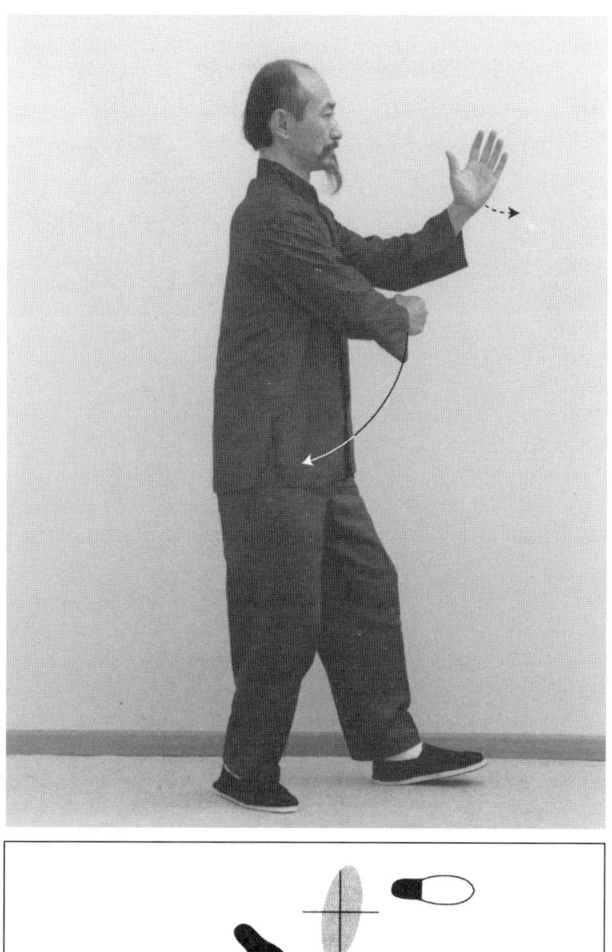

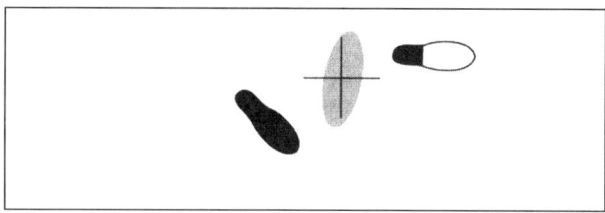

5. Turn the torso to the right until the front side of the torso faces NWW. The left leg follows the movement of the torso in a small, inward-turned arch forward (W), and then lightly place the heel (T-Step). Simultaneously, lift the left arm forward and upward at the side of the body, bend the arm, and release in the elbow while doing this until the fingertips point upward.

Lower the right arm in a small arch in front of the body and close the hand into a fist at the same time. The fist is now under the right elbow.

The front side of the torso faces NWW. You face W.

90 percent of the weight rests on the back right foot and 10 percent on the front left foot.

You are in the position "Fist under Elbow."

19. Step Back and Repulse Monkey, Right

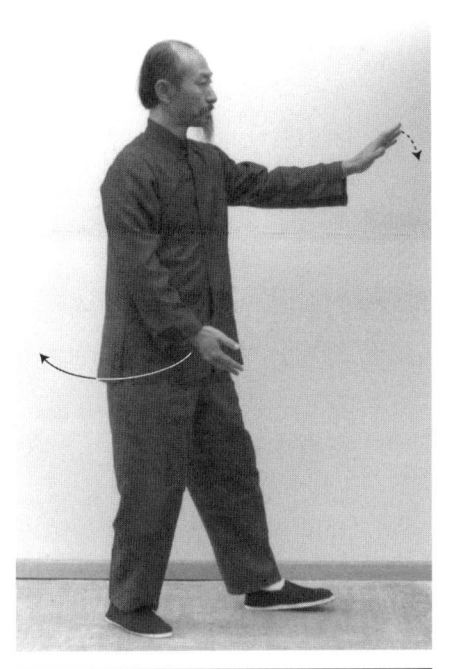

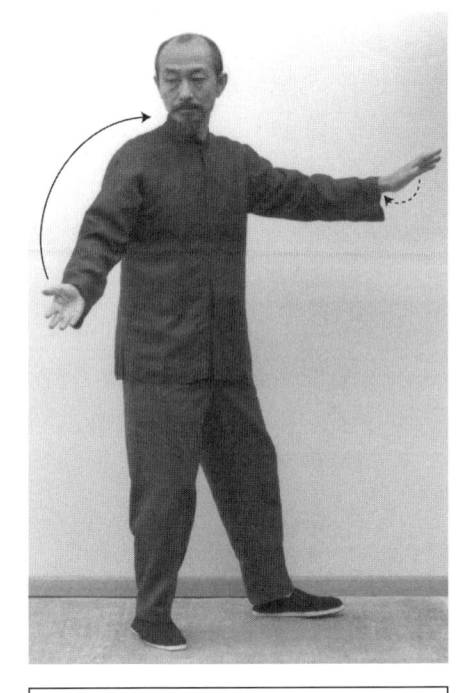

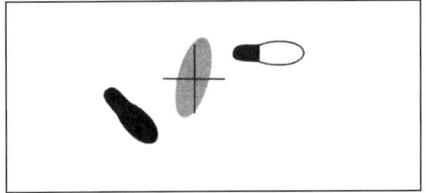

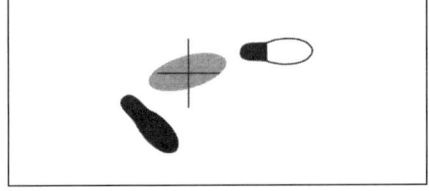

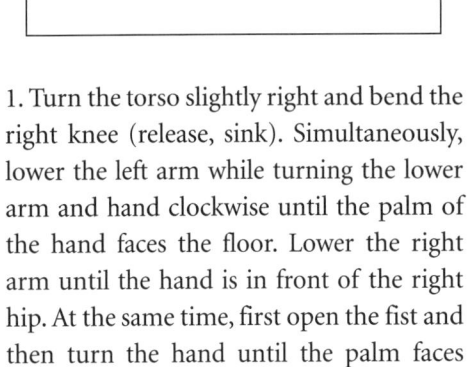

1. Turn the torso slightly right and bend the right knee (release, sink). Simultaneously, lower the left arm while turning the lower arm and hand clockwise until the palm of the hand faces the floor. Lower the right arm until the hand is in front of the right hip. At the same time, first open the fist and then turn the hand until the palm faces upward.

2. The weight stays on the right foot. Then turn the torso right until the front side faces NNW. At the same time, lift the right arm, following an arch to the NEE. Extend the left arm somewhat forward (W).

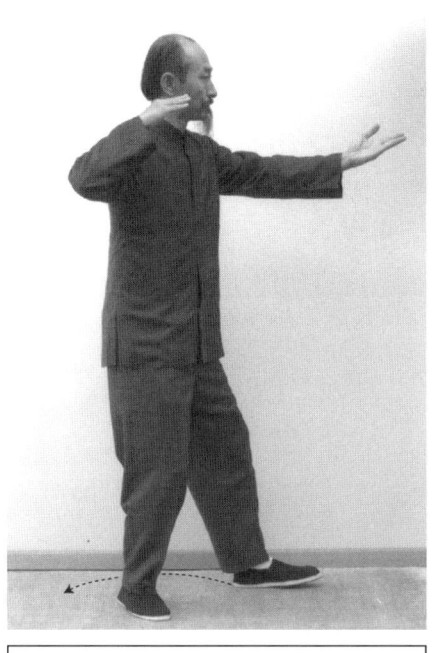

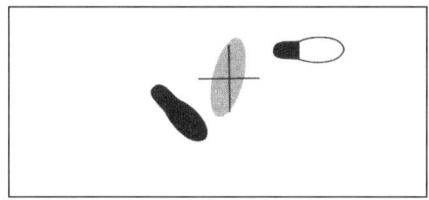

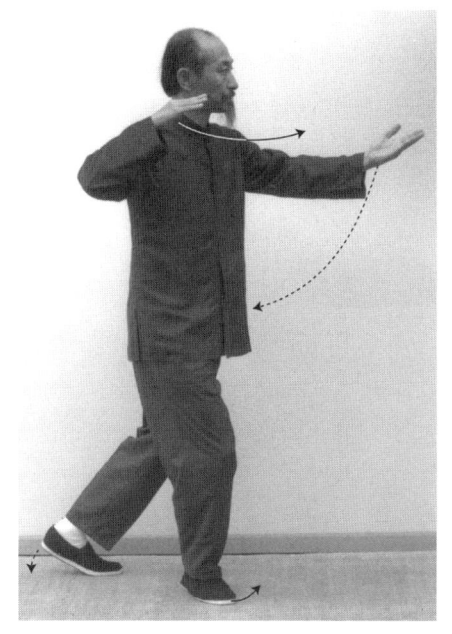

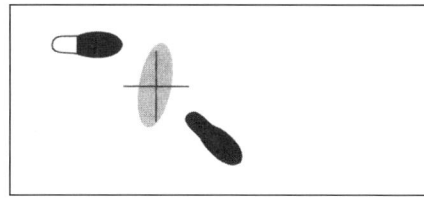

3. The weight remains on the right foot. Turn the torso left until the front side faces NWW. At the same time, turn the left lower arm and hand counterclockwise until the palm faces upward. Lift the right arm that continues to follow an arch to shoulder level and, by bending the arm, guide the hand forward until it is at neck level.

4. Place the left leg directly backward on the front part of the foot.

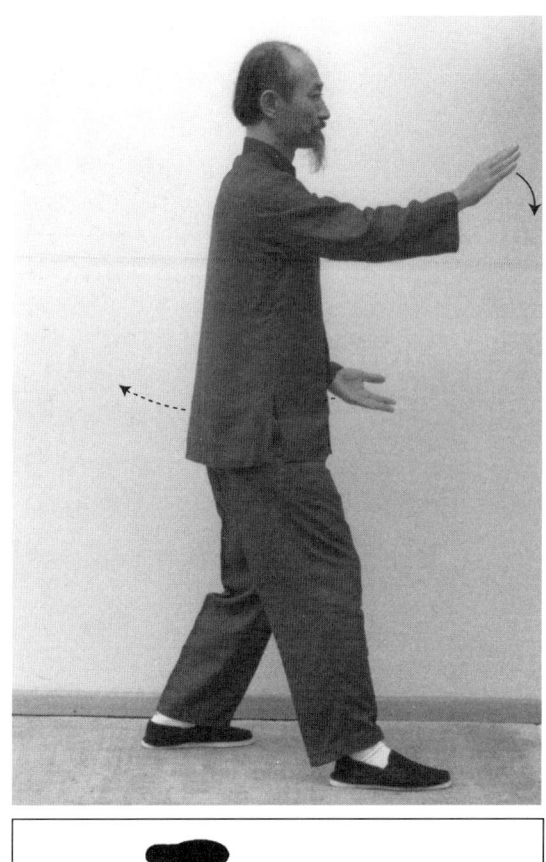

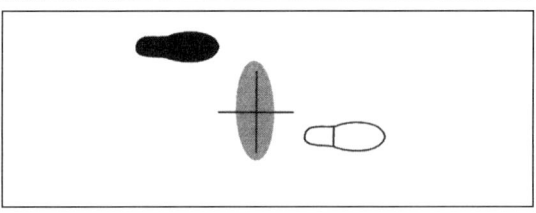

5. Turn the torso to the left until the front side faces W. At the same time, shift up to 90 percent of the weight onto the left foot, sink the foot, and bend the knee (release in the left groin fold area). Toward the end of the movement, turn the right foot on the heel to the left until the toes point W.

The arms follow the movement of the torso. Guide the right arm forward and bend the hand somewhat (standing hand) at the end of the movement. The hand indicates a push. Lower the left arm to the side of the body until the hand is in front of the left hip, the palm facing upward.

The back left foot holds 90 percent of the weight, the front right foot 10 percent.

You are in the position "Step Back and Repulse Monkey, Right."

Note: The movements demonstrated in photos 3–5 would be performed at the same time in the application (self-defense). This also applies to "Step Back and Repulse the Monkey, Left."

20. Step Back and Repulse Monkey, Left

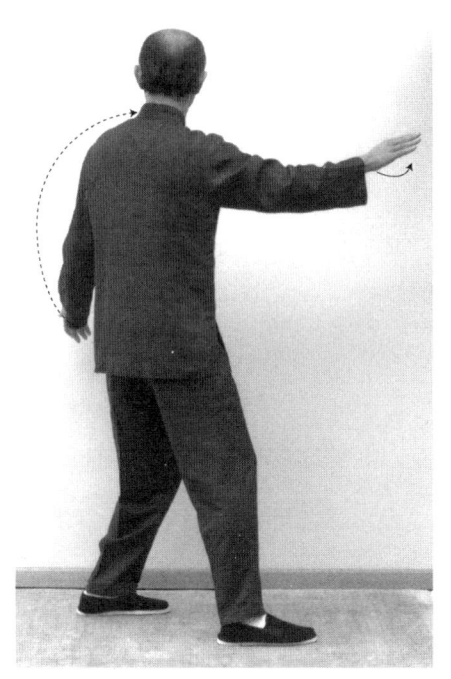

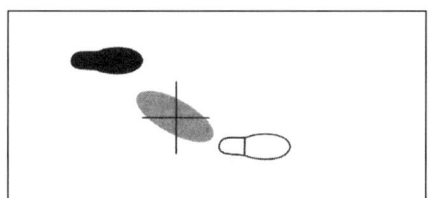

1. Turn the torso to the left until the front side faces SSW. At the same time, lift the left arm following an arch to the SEE. Extend the right arm slightly forward (W) (see position 19, photo 2).

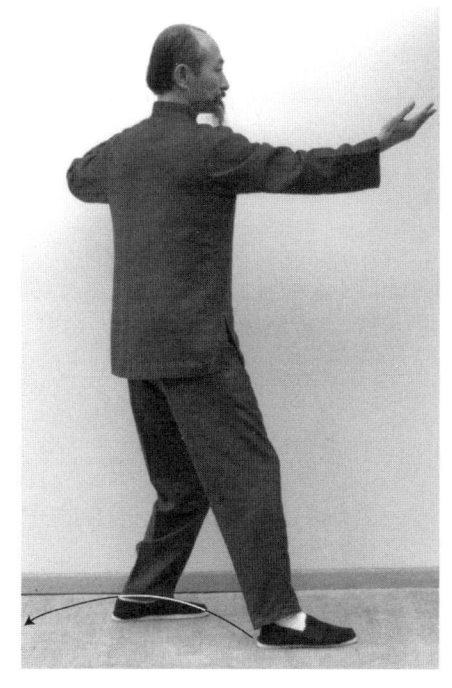

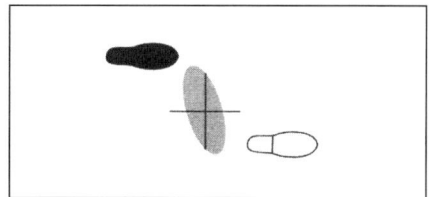

2. The weight stays on the left foot. Turn the torso to the right until the front side faces SWW. While doing so, turn the right lower arm and hand clockwise until the palm of the hand faces upward. Lift the left arm following an arch to shoulder height and guide the hand forward by bending the arm. The hand is at neck level.

3. Place the right leg directly backward on the front part of the foot.*

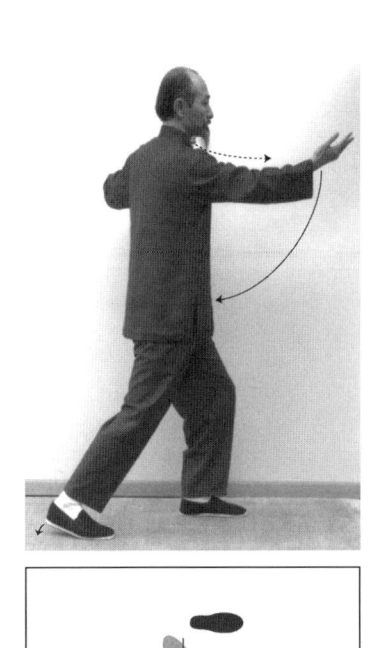

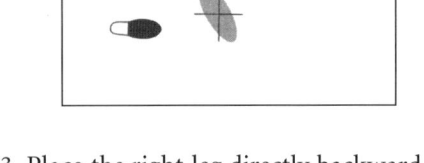

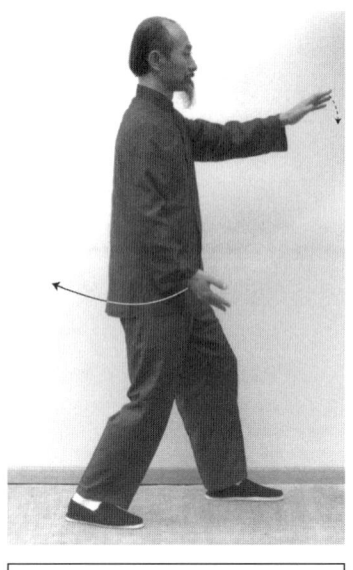

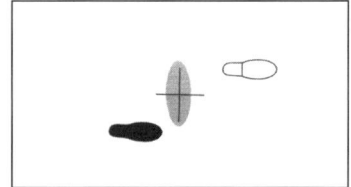

4. Turn the torso to the right until the front side faces W. At the same time, shift up to 90 percent of the weight onto the right foot, sink the foot, and bend the knee (release in the right groin fold). The arms follow the movement of the torso. Guide the left arm forward and toward the end of the movement slightly bend the hand (standing hand). The hand indicates a push. Lower the right arm to the side of the body until the hand is in front of the right hip with the palm of the hand facing upward.

90 percent of the weight rests on the back right foot and 10 percent on the front left foot.

You are in the position "Step Back and Repulse Monkey, Left."

* Cheng Man-Ch'ing found it very important that the feet were placed parallel in "Step Back and Repulse Monkey." This step system is adopted from the Chen-style. In the old Yang-style, however, a step similar to the Bow Step is used in "Step Back and Repulse Monkey."

Repetition

Step Back and Repulse Monkey, Right (19)*

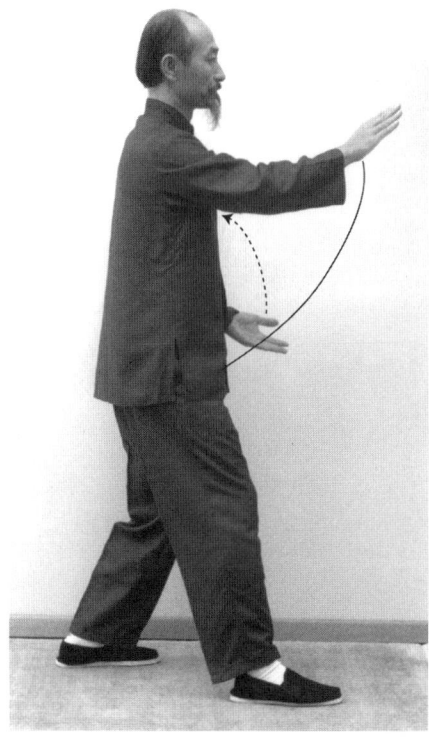

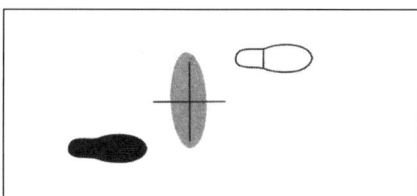

You are in the position "Step Back and Repulse Monkey, Right."†

---

* The Repulse Monkey can also be performed five times instead of three times.
† Repulse Monkey is especially used against Hsing I attacks because its techniques employ steps that follow direct lines forward and backward.

21. Diagonal Flying

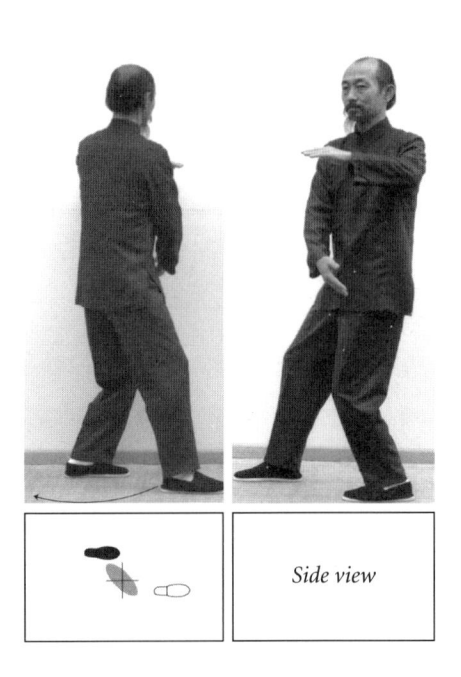

Side view

1. Turn the torso to the left until the front side faces SW. Simultaneously, lower the right arm until the hand is in front of the left hip with the palm of the hand turned upward. Lift the left arm (hand in front of the central axis). As you do this, turn the hand until the palm of the hand faces downward.

Not shown: Turn the torso to the right until the front side faces NWW. The arms follow the movement of the torso without changing their position.

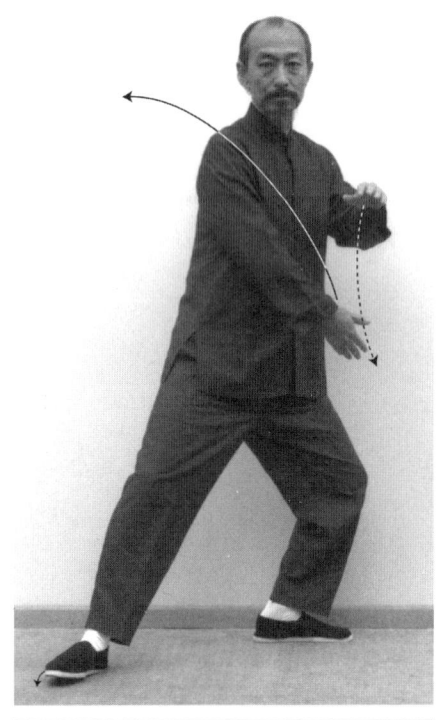

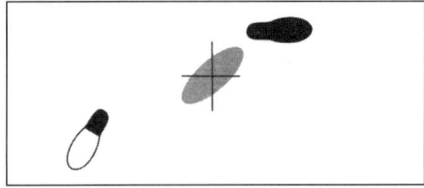

2. Turn the torso to the right until the front side faces NW. At the same time, place the right leg with the heel to the NE.

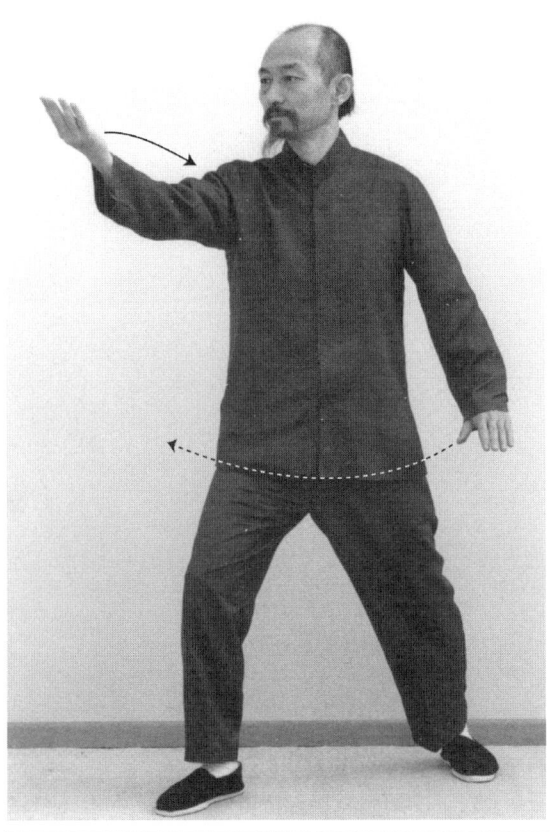

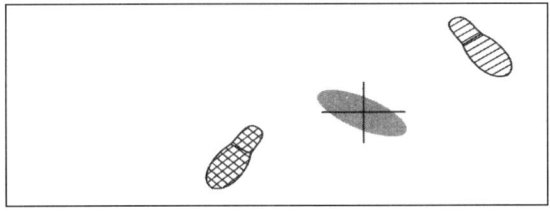

3. Turn the torso and the left leg on the heel to the right until the front side faces NNE and the toes of the left foot point NNW (Millstone Principle, Bow Step). While doing so, shift up to 70 percent of the weight onto the right foot and sink the foot (the toes point 30° away from direct N), and bend the knee. Lift the right arm upward and forward, following a big arch until the right palm faces upward. Lower the left arm to the side of the body and bring it slightly outward. Toward the end of the movement, bend the hand (standing hand).

The front side of the torso faces NNE.

70 percent of the weight rests on the front right foot and 30 percent on the back left foot.

You are in the position "Diagonal Flying."

22. Wave Hands in Clouds, Left

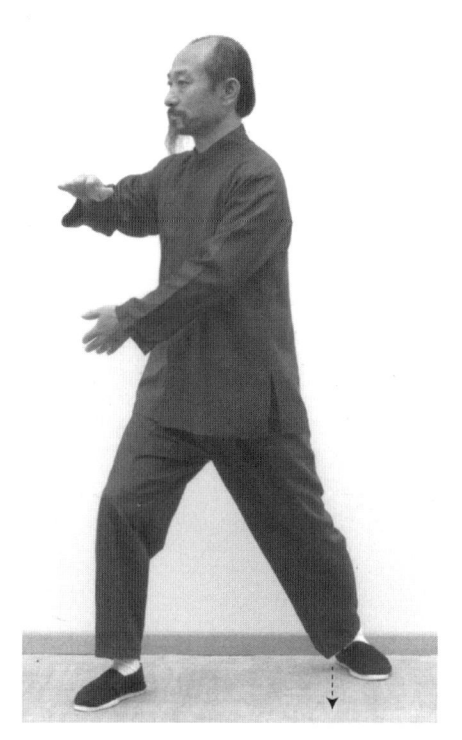

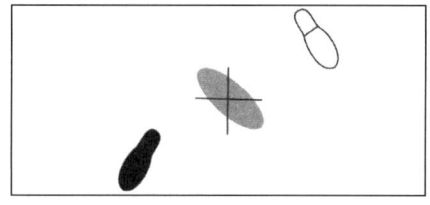

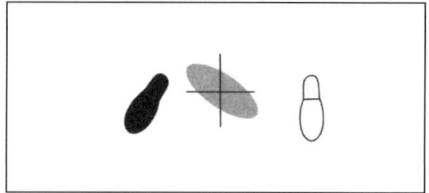

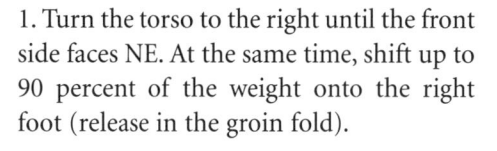

1. Turn the torso to the right until the front side faces NE. At the same time, shift up to 90 percent of the weight onto the right foot (release in the groin fold).

Simultaneously, pull the right arm to the right side of the body. Bend the arm while turning the lower arm and hand counterclockwise until the palm of the hand faces downward.

Guide the left arm to the right until the hand is in front of the right hip with its palm turned upward. Both hands are now in a fall-line.

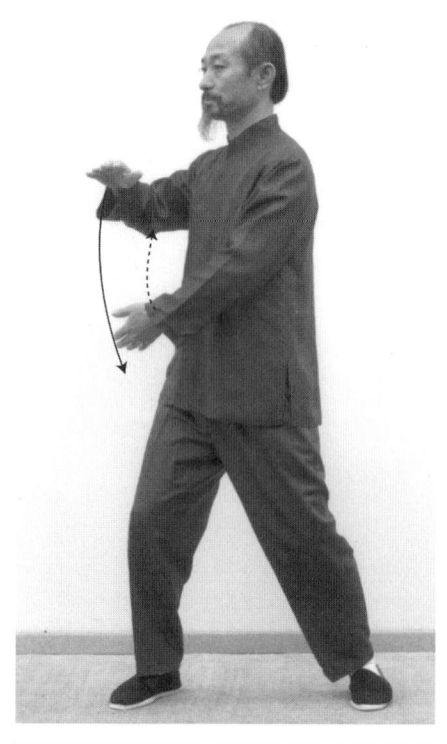

2. Place the left leg, with the heel first, forward (N).

The toes point to the N.

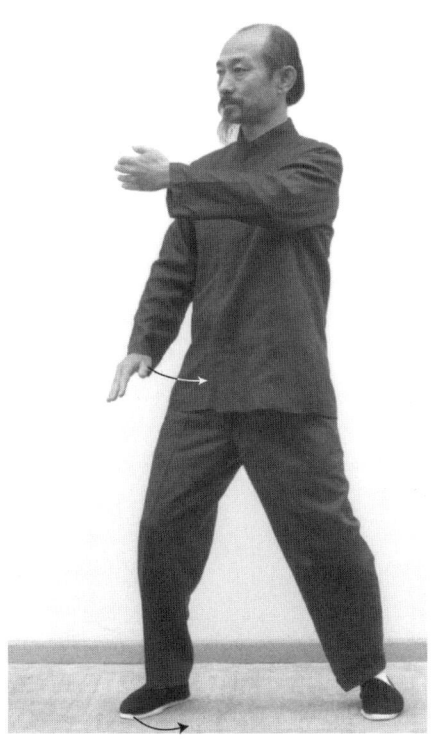

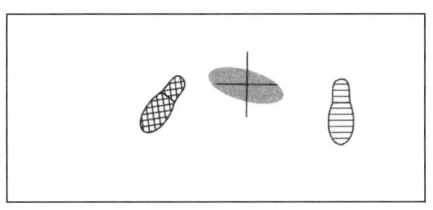

3. Turn the torso to the left until the front side faces NNE (Millstone Principle). At the same time, shift up to 30 percent of the weight onto the left foot. Lower the right arm at the side of the body. Toward the end of this movement, turn the lower arm and hand until the palm of the hand faces the body. Simultaneously, lift the left arm in front of the body with the palm of the hand facing the body (Ward-Off).

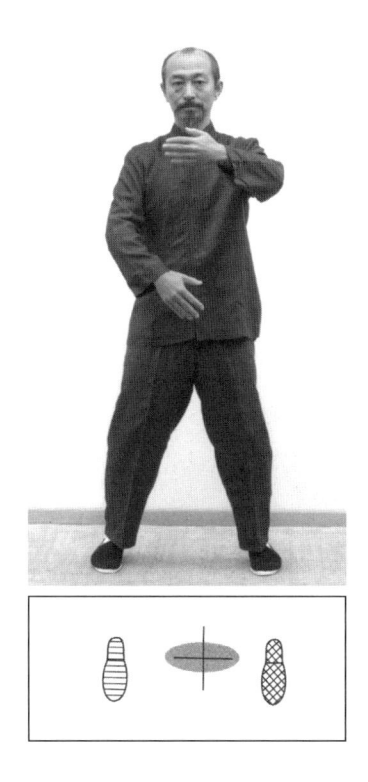

4. Turn the torso to the left until the front side faces N. While doing so, shift up to 70 percent of the weight onto the left foot. Accompany the torso turn by turning the right foot left on the heel until the toes point N (Large Parallel Stance).

The arms follow the movement of the torso. Guide the right arm to the left until the hand is in front of the central axis (Ward-Off). The position of the left arm stays the same (Ward-Off).

70 percent of the weight rests on the left foot and 30 percent on the right foot.

You are in the position "Wave Hands in Clouds, Left."*

* Wave Hands in Clouds, Left: The movement sequence to the *left*, *left* arm on top, 70 percent of your weight on the *left* foot.

23. Wave Hands in Clouds, Right

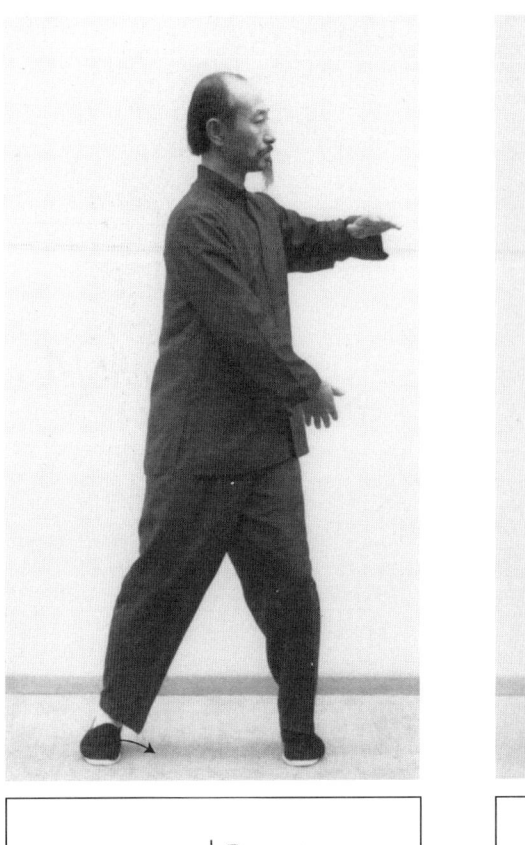

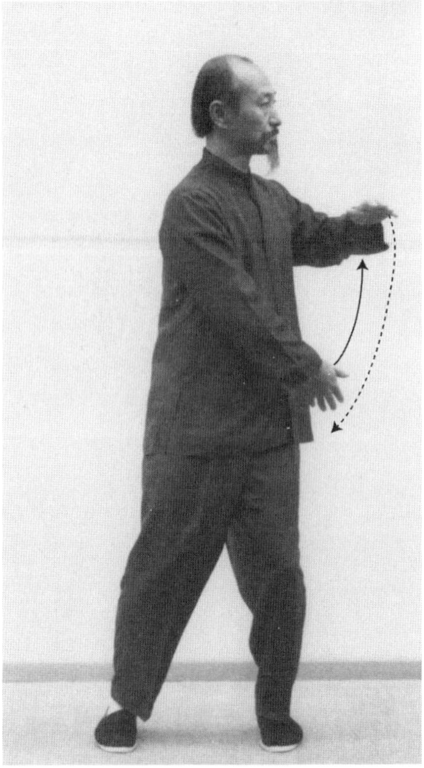

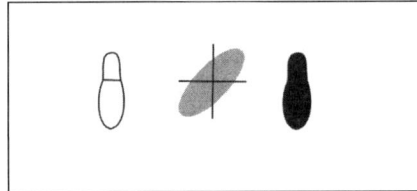

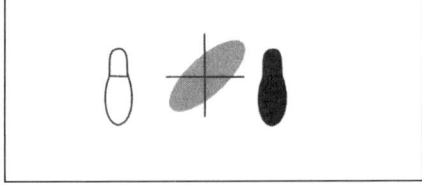

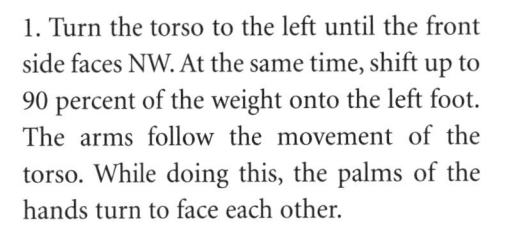

1. Turn the torso to the left until the front side faces NW. At the same time, shift up to 90 percent of the weight onto the left foot. The arms follow the movement of the torso. While doing this, the palms of the hands turn to face each other.

2. Place the right leg to the left (Parallel Stance). Place the inner edge of the foot down first.

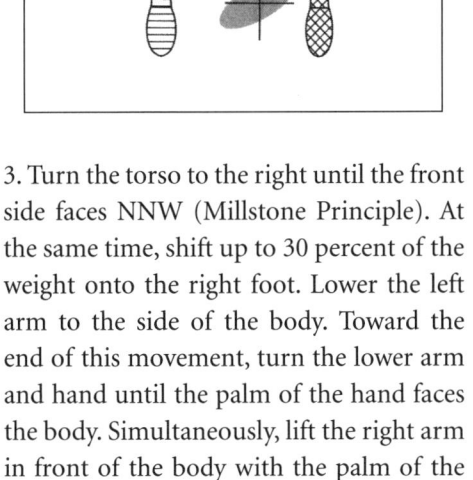

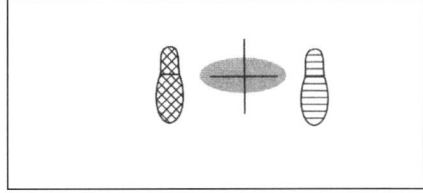

3. Turn the torso to the right until the front side faces NNW (Millstone Principle). At the same time, shift up to 30 percent of the weight onto the right foot. Lower the left arm to the side of the body. Toward the end of this movement, turn the lower arm and hand until the palm of the hand faces the body. Simultaneously, lift the right arm in front of the body with the palm of the hand facing the body (Ward-Off).

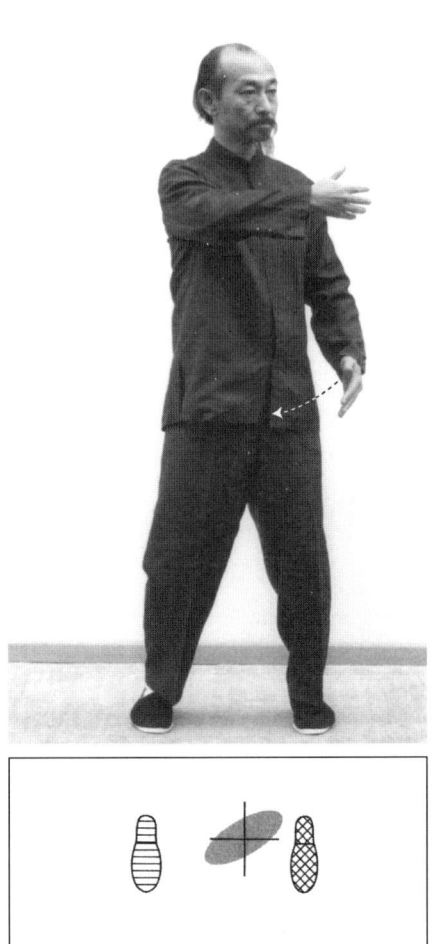

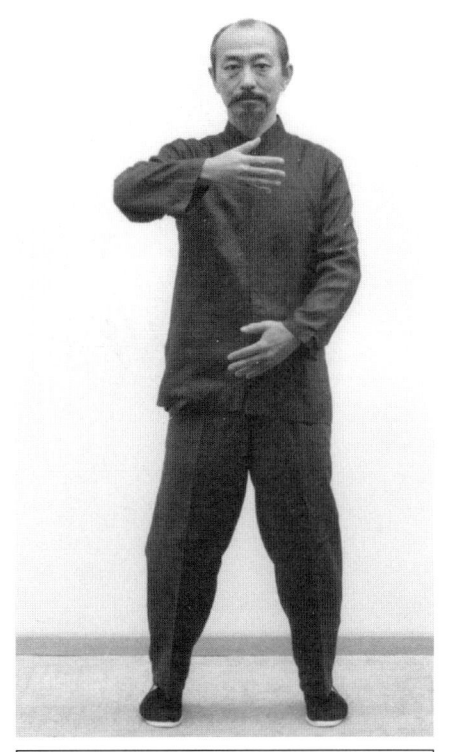

4. Turn the torso to the right until the front side faces N. While doing so, shift up to 70 percent of the weight onto the right foot. The arms follow the movement of the torso. Guide the left arm to the right until the hand is in front of the central axis (Ward-Off). The right arm's position stays the same (Ward-Off).

70 percent of the weight rests on the right foot and 30 percent on the left foot.

You are in the position "Wave Hands in Clouds, Right."

Repetition

1. Wave Hands in Clouds, Left (22)*

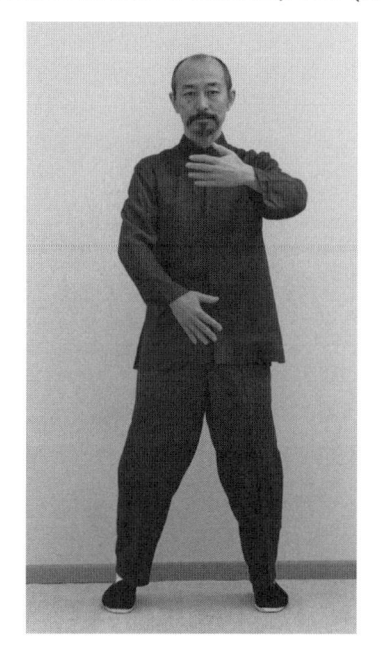

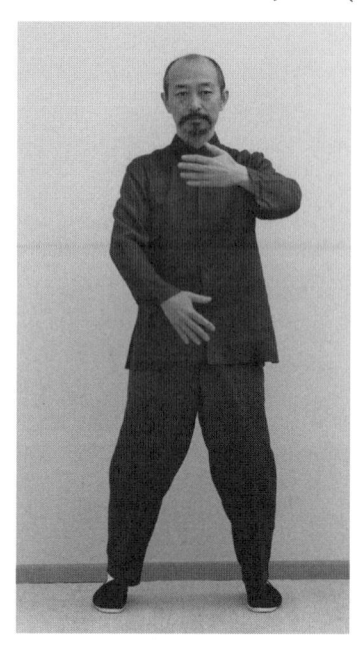

2. Wave Hands in Clouds, Right (23)

3. Wave Hands in Clouds, Left (22)*

You are in the position "Wave Hands in Clouds, Left."

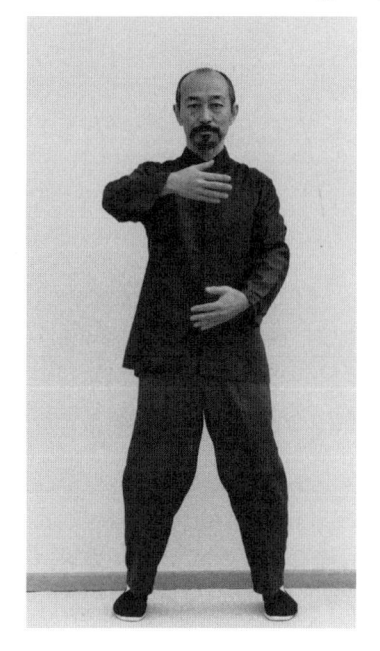

* Step without turning the foot, Parallel Stance.

Single Whip (8)

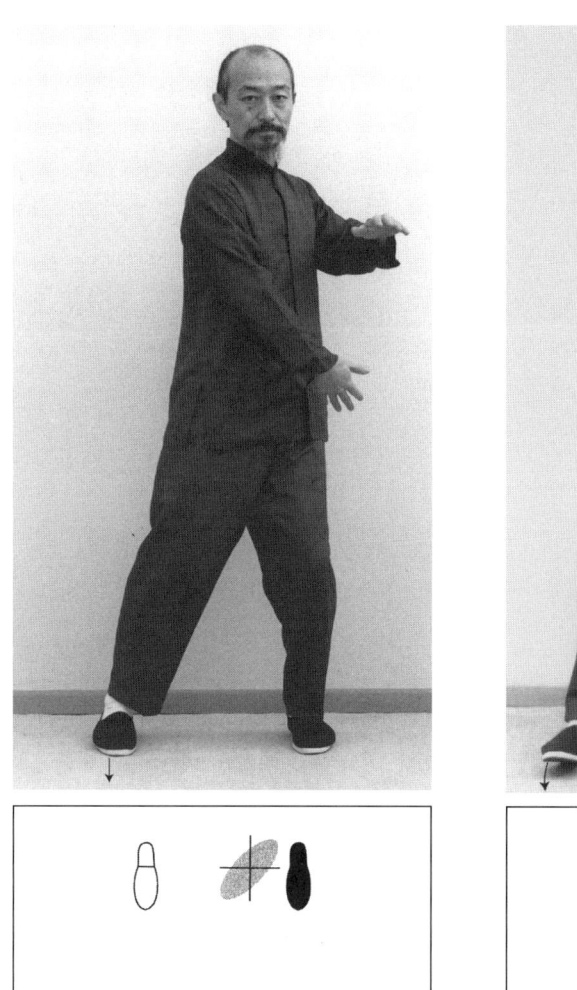

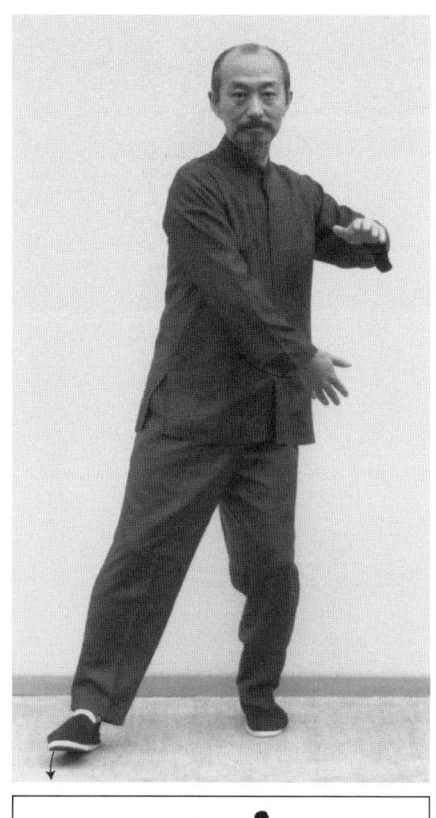

1. Turn the torso to the left until the front side faces NW. At the same time, shift up to 90 percent of your weight onto the left foot. Simultaneously, pull the left arm to the left side of the body. Bend the arm and, at the same time, turn the lower arm and hand clockwise until the palm of the hand faces downward. Guide the right arm to the left until the hand is in front of the left hip; as you do this, turn the palm of the hand upward. Both hands are now in a fall-line. You look forward.

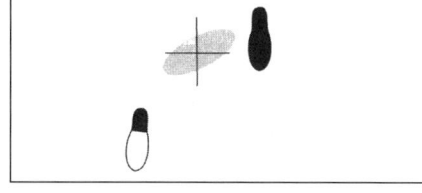

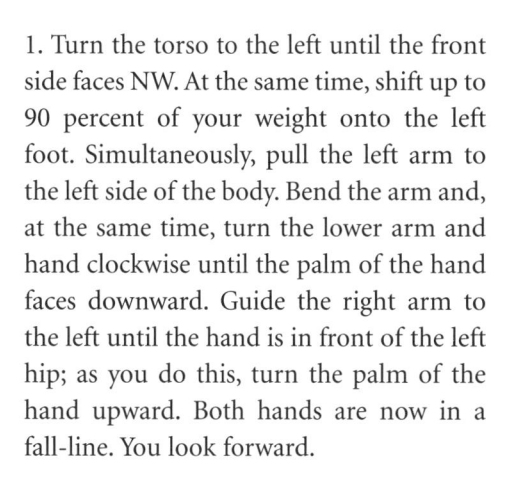

2. Turn the torso to the right until the front side faces NNW. At the same time, place the right leg forward (N) with the heel. The toes point N.

The arms remain in the same positions as they follow the movement of the torso.

3. Shift up to 70 percent of the weight onto the right foot, sink the foot, and bend the knee. Simultaneously, bend the right arm, first raising it with the elbow NE (elbow strike). Slightly sink the left arm.

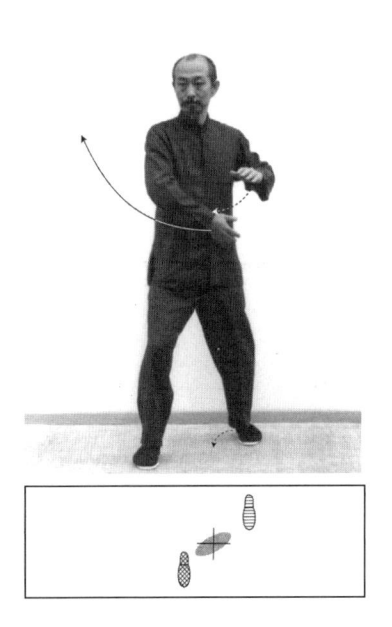

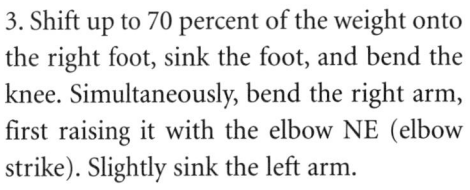

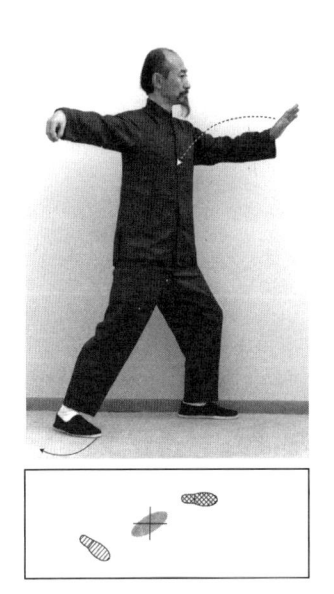

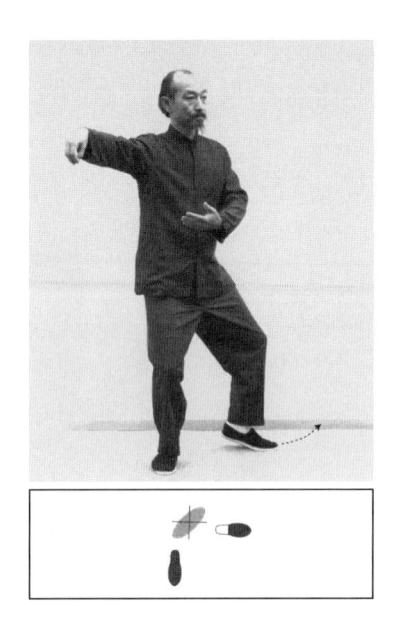

4. Turn the torso to the left until the front side faces NW. While doing this, shift up to 90 percent of the weight onto the right foot. The left leg, heel raised, follows the torso until the toes point W. As the torso turns, stretch the right arm to the NE. (Don't completely stretch out the arm!) At the same time, bend the hand and close the fingers into a "bird's head." Slightly sink the left arm and bring it closer to the body. The palm of the hand turns to the body (Ward-Off).

You repeat the position "Single Whip." (See position 8, photos 5–7.)

24. Squatting Single Whip

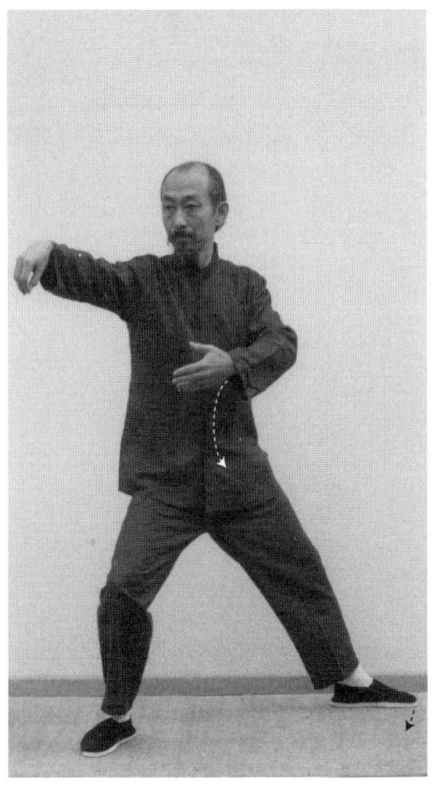

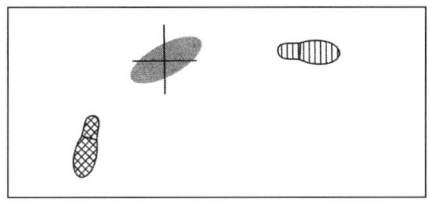

1. Turn the torso to the right until the front side faces NNW. At the same time, shift up to 70 percent of the weight onto the right foot. Accompany the torso turn by turning the right leg on the heel to the right until the toes point NNE. Simultaneously, guide the left lower arm and hand as one unit in front of the body until the hand is in front of the breastbone. While doing this, turn the palm of the hand toward the body (Ward-Off).

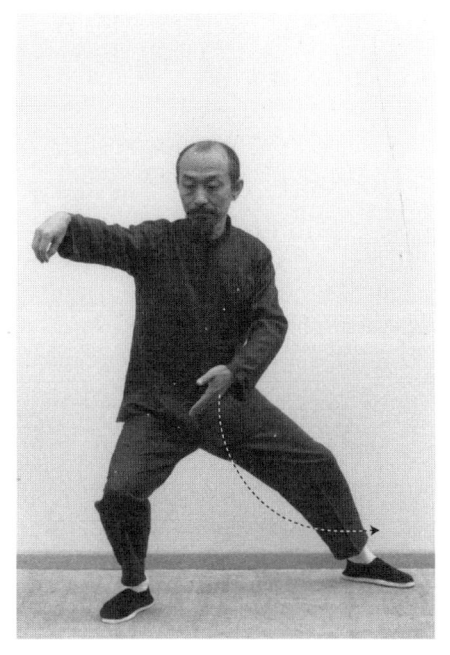

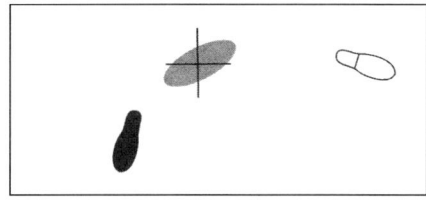

2. Turn the torso to the left until the front side faces NW. At the same time, shift up to 90 percent of the weight onto the right foot and bend the knee. Accompany the weight shift by turning the left foot on the heel somewhat inward, until the toes point NWW.

Simultaneously, lower the left arm in a clockwise arch in front of the body. The position of the right arm stays the same.

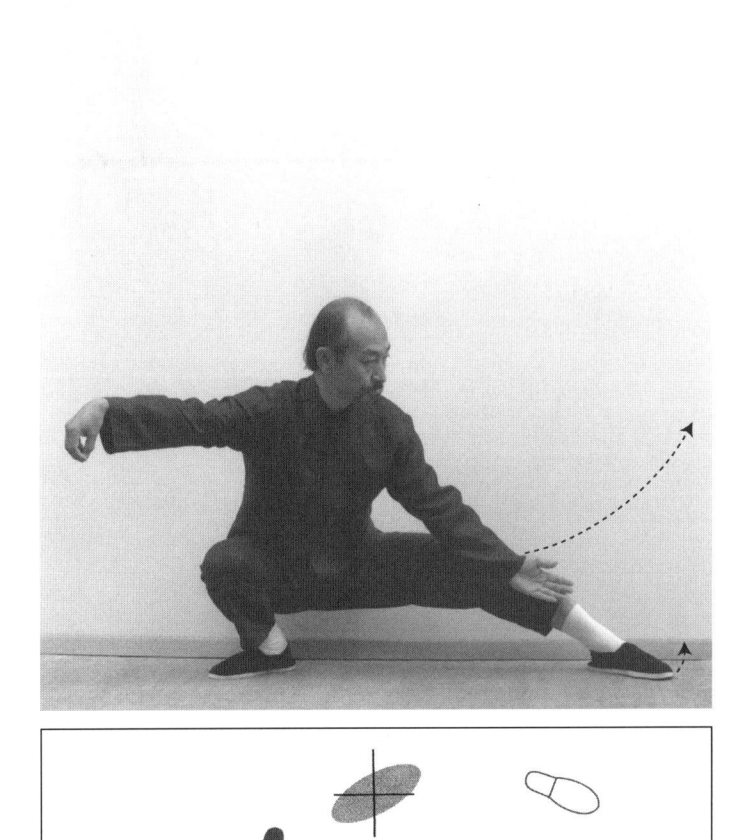

3. Crouch down, keeping the posture as straight as possible. Toward the end of this movement, through a slight hip turn to the left, guide the left arm forward following an arch. The position of the right arm stays the same.

The front of the torso faces NW. You look to the W.

90 percent of the weight rests on the back right foot and 10 percent on the front left foot.

You are in the position "Squatting Single Whip."

Note: This position is easier to perform if one takes a Bow Step that is longer than normal.

25. Golden Cock Stands on One Leg, Right

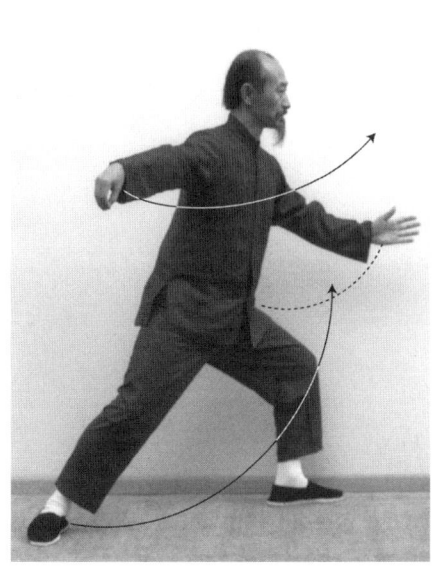

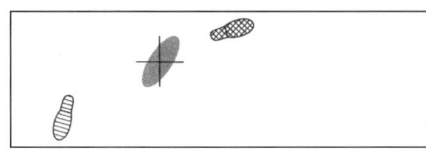

1. Turn the torso to the left until the front side faces NWW. At the same time, shift up to 70 percent of the weight onto the front left leg. While doing this torso turn, the left foot turns to the left without being raised (the toes point 30° away from direct W).

Simultaneously, lift the left arm forward and upward following an arch. Slightly lower the right arm.

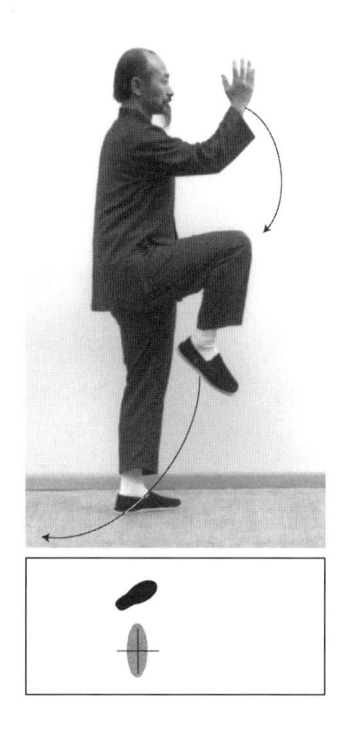

2. a) Turn the torso to the left until the front side faces W. While doing this, shift all the weight onto the left foot. Pull the right leg forward and bend it. Simultaneously, guide the right arm forward and upward following an arch while turning the hand clockwise and opening the "Bird's Head." The position of the left arm stays the same.

b) Stretch the left leg somewhat while raising the bent right leg in front of the body (allow the lower leg and foot to hang freely and relaxed). Simultaneously, bend the right arm until the fingertips point upward. Lower the left arm to the side of the body. Toward the end of this movement, bend the hand slightly (standing hand).

See page 146 for a side view.

The weight rests on the left foot.

You are in the position "Golden Cock Stands on One Leg, Right."

26. Golden Cock Stands on One Leg, Left

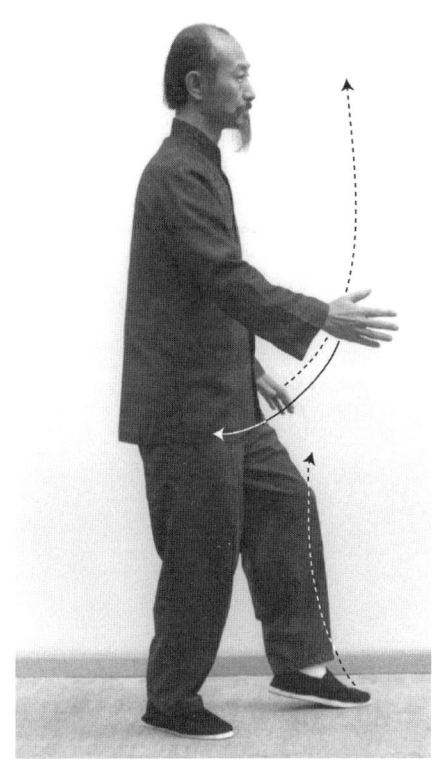

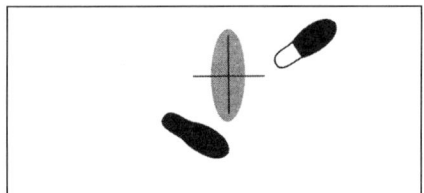

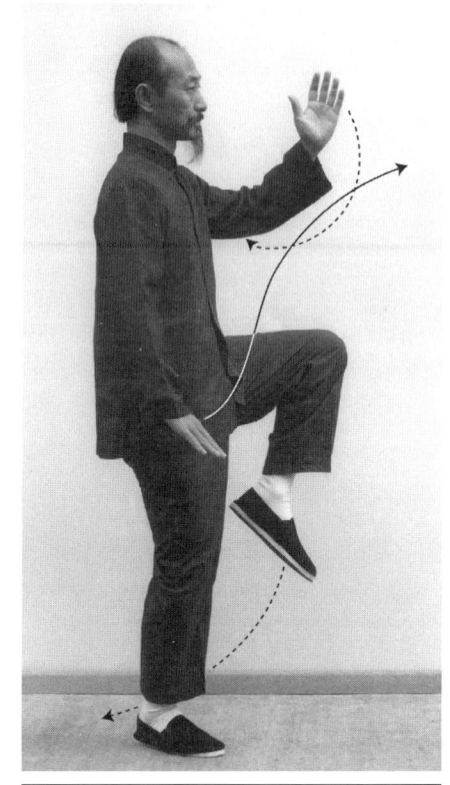

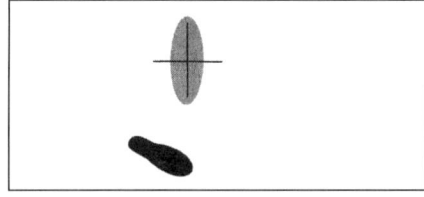

Not shown: Slightly bend the left knee. Sink the right leg and place it behind you, setting down the front part of the foot first. The toes point 30° away from direct W.

1. Shift up to 90 percent of the weight onto the right foot; bend the knee. Slightly lift the heel of the left foot. At the same time, lower the right arm to the side of the body and lift the left arm somewhat.

2. Stretch the right leg somewhat while lifting the left leg and the left arm. When lifting the left arm, the hand (palm of the hand faces toward the body), is first raised in front of the central axis and then brought upward and to the left until the fingertips point upward. Lower the right arm to the side of the body; toward the end of this movement bend the hand somewhat (standing hand).

The weight rests on the right foot.

You are in the position "Golden Cock Stands on One Leg, Left."

27. Separate Right Foot

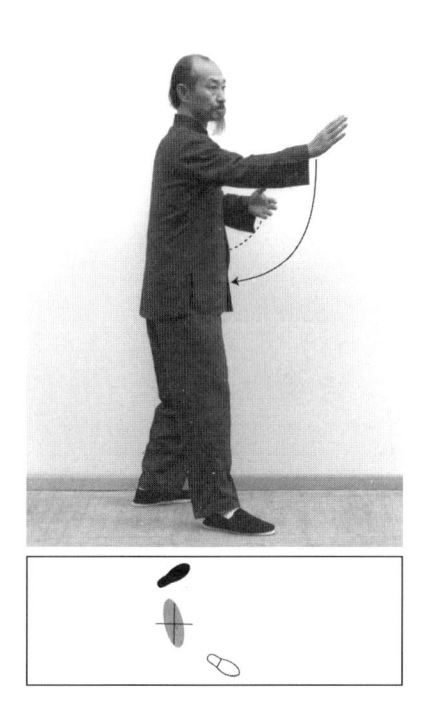

1. a) Slightly bend the right knee. At the same time, turn the torso SWW and place the left leg backward, setting down the inner edge of the foot first. The toes point 30° away from direct W.

b) Shift up to 90 percent of the weight onto the left foot, and bend the knee. Accompany the torso turn and the weight shift by raising the right arm. While doing so, first raise the hand with the palm of the hand turned to the body following an arch in front of the central axis and then bring it upward and forward (NW). Simultaneously, lower the left arm and hand in front of the central axis. At the same time, turn the lower arm and hand counterclockwise until the palm of the hand points upward.*

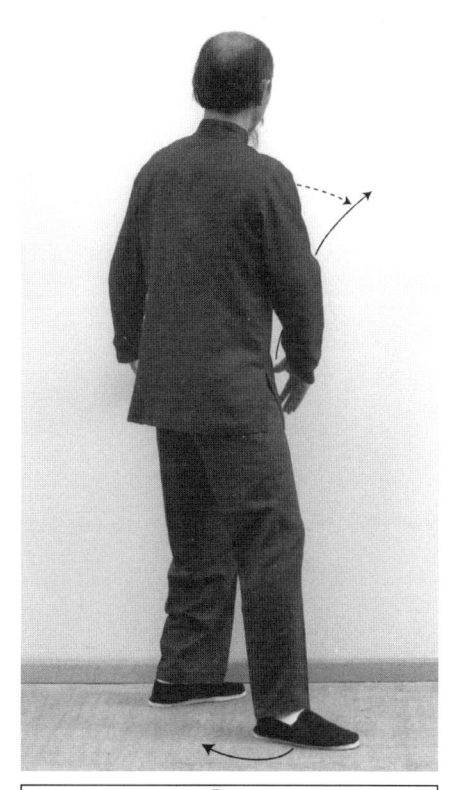

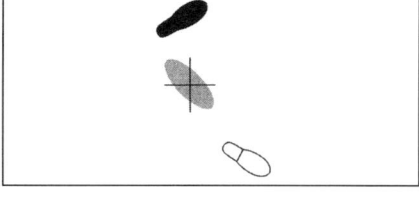

2. Turn the torso to the left until the front side faces SW (release and sink). Both arms follow the movement of the torso to the left and are lowered following arches.

*This sequence of movements contains the technique "High Pat on Horse," which is an individual position in the long form of the Yang-style.

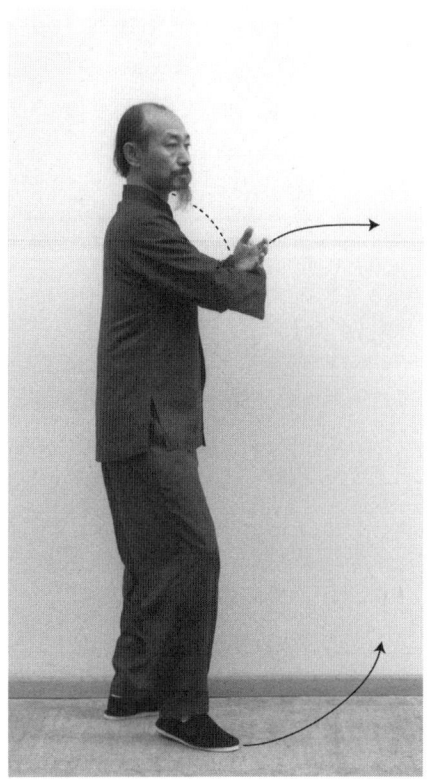

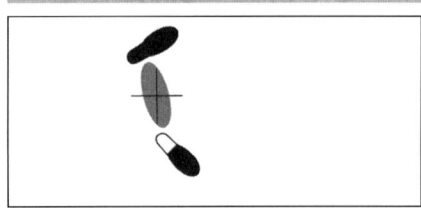

3. Turn the torso to the right until the front side faces WSW. While doing so, lift the arms in arching movement and bring them together in front of the body (breastbone) until the wrists cross. The palms of the hands face the body with the right hand on the outside. As you turn the torso, lift the right leg and place it somewhat closer to the body, setting down the front part of the foot. The toes now point NW.

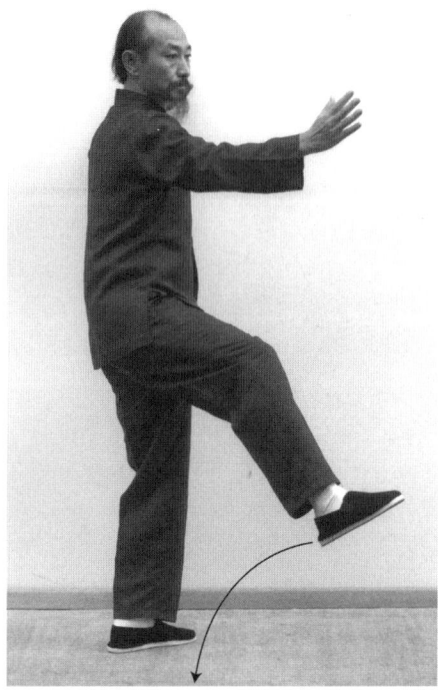

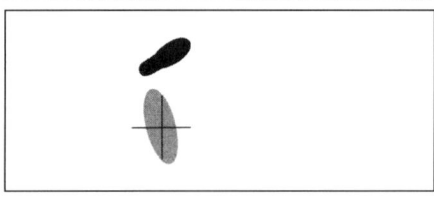

4. Stretch the left leg somewhat. At the same time, lift the right leg NW and indicate a kick with the toes. Simultaneously, separate the arms. While doing so, turn the lower arms and hands outward as one unit. Toward the end of this movement, bend both hands slightly (standing hand).*

The front side of the torso faces WSW.

You look to the NW. The weight rests on the left foot.

You are in the position "Separate Right Foot."

* Bending the left hand serves to stabilize the balance.

148

28. Separate Left Foot

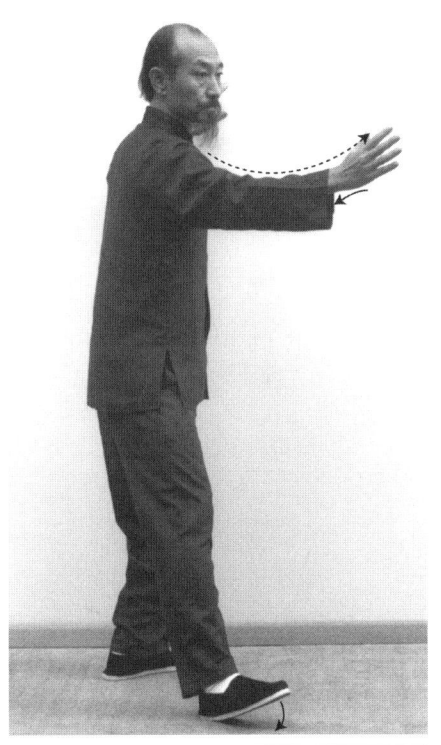

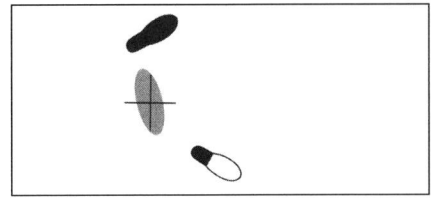

Not shown: Sink the right lower leg and foot.

1. Bend the left knee. At the same time, place the right leg NW with the heel first and the toes pointing 30° N.

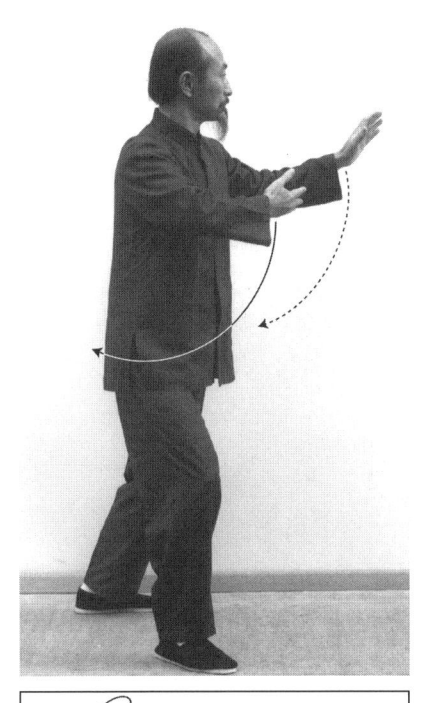

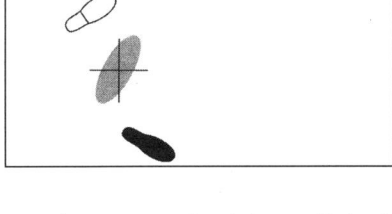

2. Turn the torso to the right until the front side faces NWW. At the same time, shift up to 90 percent of the weight onto the right foot, sink the foot, and bend the knee. The arms follow the movement of the torso. Guide the lower arm and hand of the right arm in front of the body by releasing in the elbow. While doing this, turn the lower arm and hand clockwise until the hand is in front of the central axis and the palm of the hand faces upward. Simultaneously, stretch the left arm to the SW in an inward-directed arch, fingertips first ("High Pat on Horse").

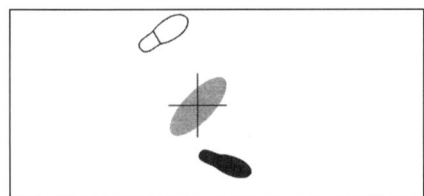

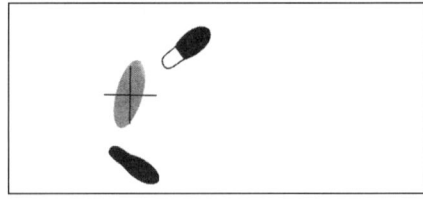

3. Turn the torso to the right until the front side faces NW (release, sink). Both arms follow the movement of the torso to the right and are lowered by following arches.

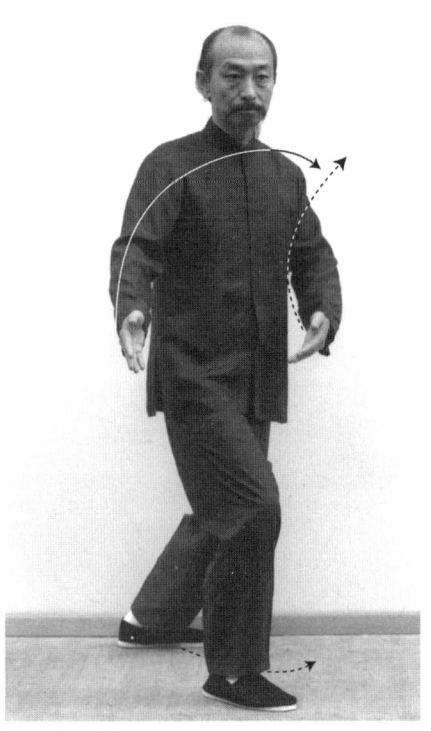

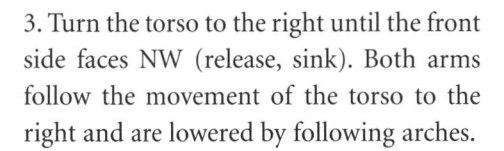

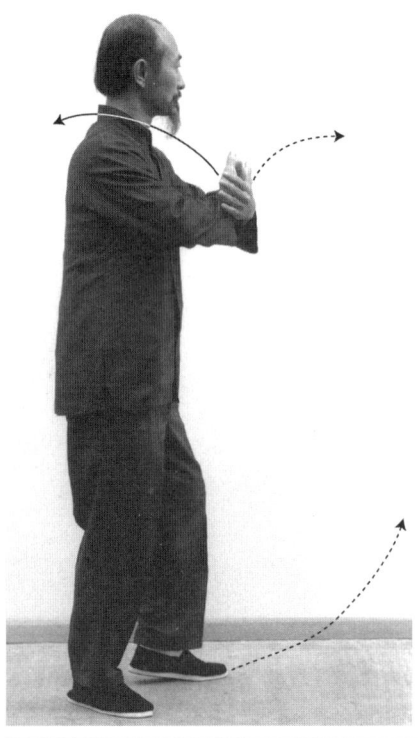

4. Turn the torso to the left until the front side faces NWW. While doing this, lift the arms farther following arches and bring them together in front of the body (breastbone) until the wrists cross. The palms of the hands face the body; the left hand is on the outside. As the torso turns, lift the left leg and place it forward on the front part of the foot. The toes point SW.

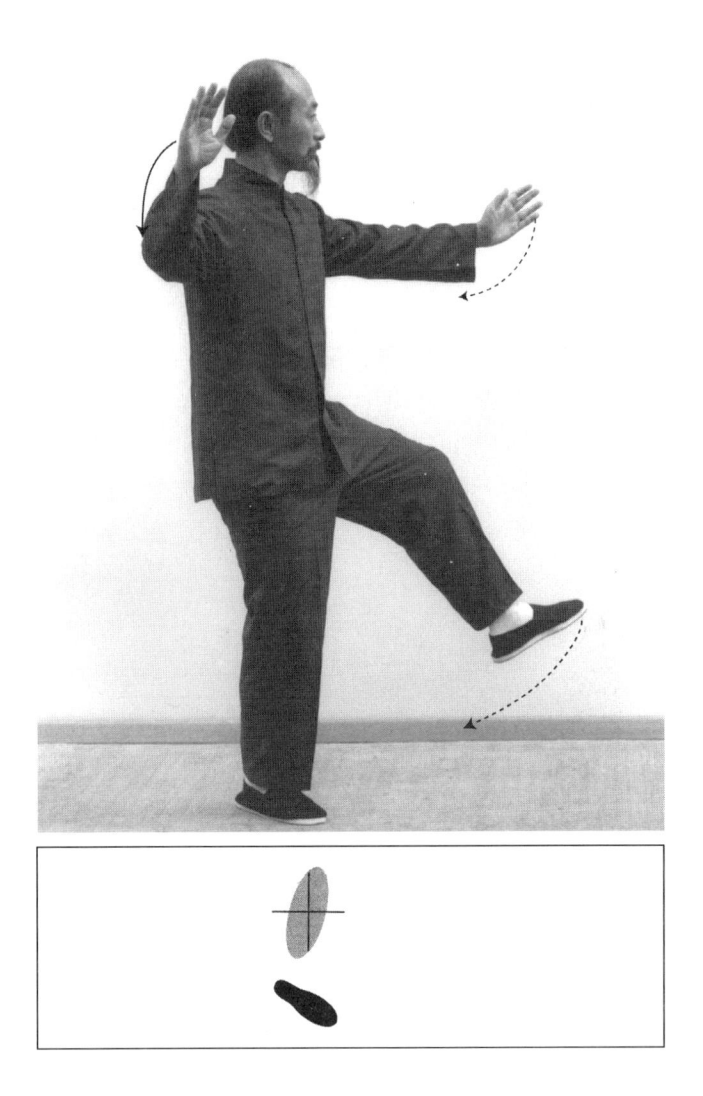

5. Stretch the right leg somewhat. At the same time, lift the left leg to the SW and indicate a kick with the toes. Simultaneously, open the arms and move them apart. While doing this, turn the lower arms and hands outward as one unit. Toward the end of this movement, slightly bend the hands (standing hand).*

The front side of the torso faces NWW. You look SW.

The weight rests on the right foot.

You are in the position "Separate Left Foot."

* Bending the right hand serves to stabilize the balance.

29. Turn and Kick with Left Heel

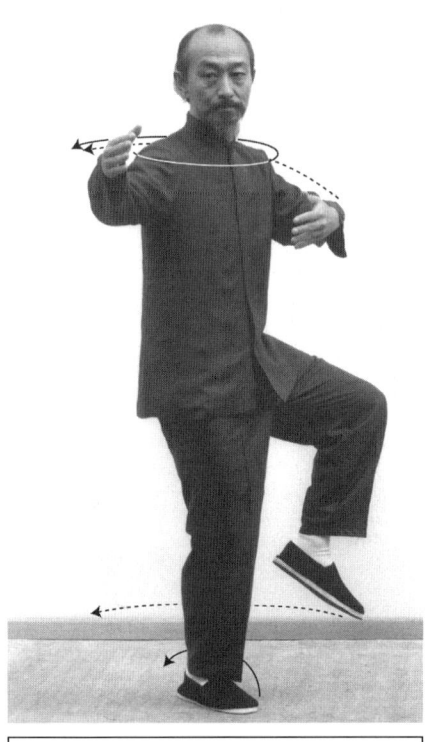

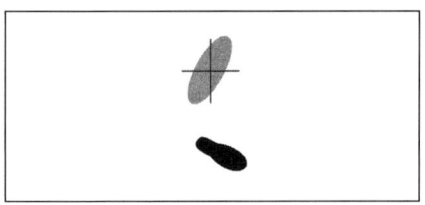

1. a) Sink the left lower leg and foot.

b) Turn the torso slightly to the right. The left leg follows the movement of the torso until the knee faces W. The arms follow the movement of the torso. Guide the left lower arm and hand in front of the body until the palm of the hand is turned toward the body. Simultaneously, sink the right lower arm and hand while turning the hand slightly clockwise.

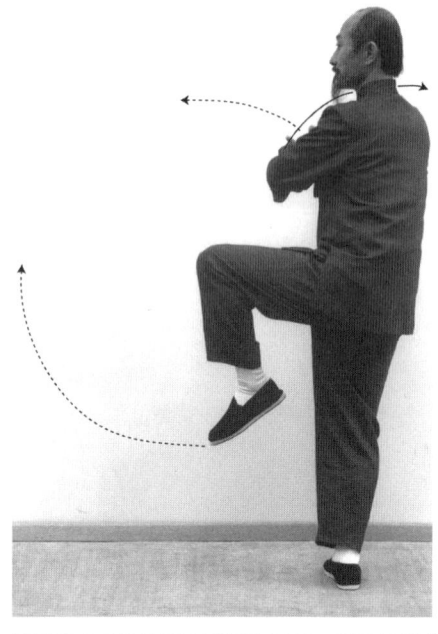

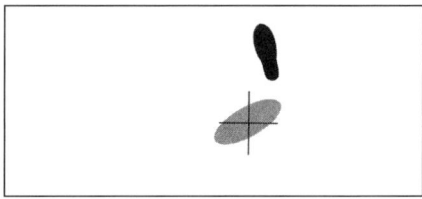

2. Turn the torso on the right heel 180° to the left until the front side faces SSE. The toes point slightly beyond S.

The left leg follows the torso turn until the knee faces E. The left arm remains in front of the body during the torso turn. Bend the right arm and guide it inward and behind the left arm until the wrists cross. The palms of the hands face the body.

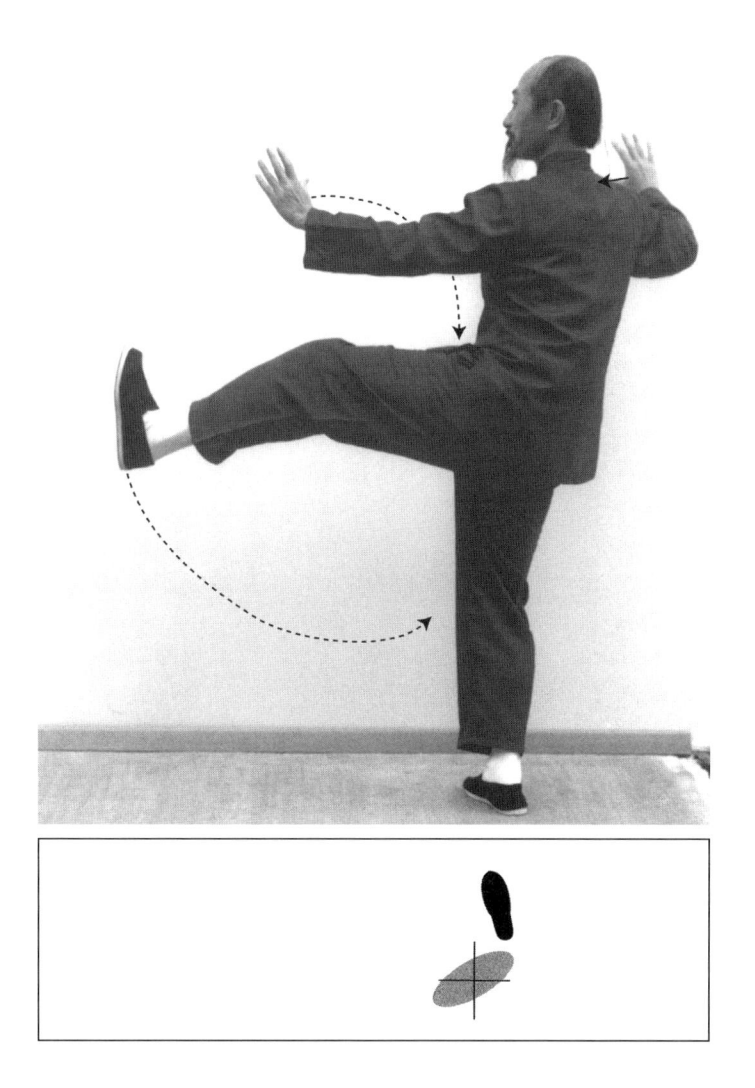

3. Stretch the right leg somewhat. At the same time, slightly lift the left thigh and then indicate a kick to the E. Simultaneously, open the arms and move them apart from each other. While doing so, turn the lower arms and hands outward as one unit. Toward the end of this movement bend both hands slightly (standing hand).

The weight rests on the right front foot.

The front side of the torso faces SEE.

You look E.

You are in the position "Turn and Kick with Left Heel."

Repetition

Brush Left-Knee—Twist Step (12)

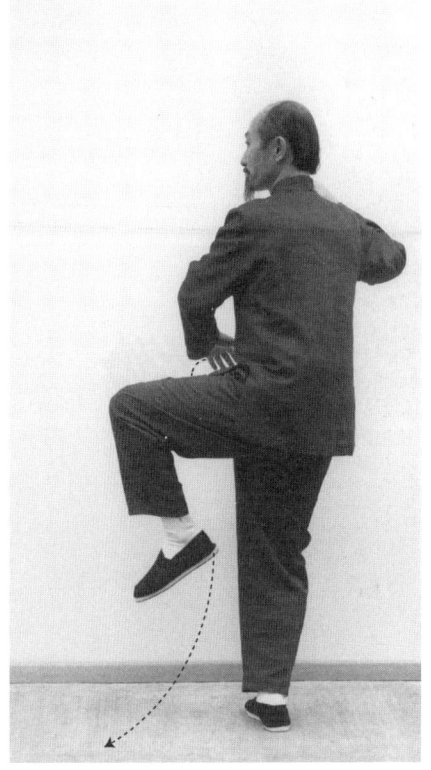

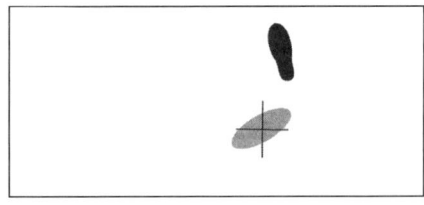

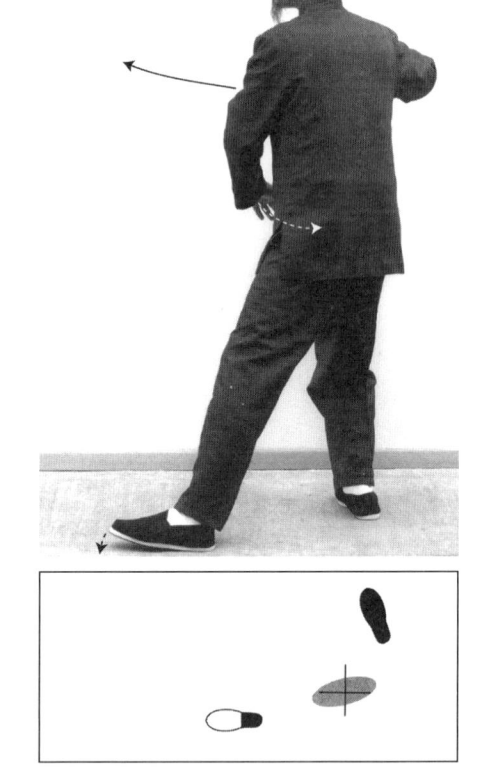

1. Slightly bend the right knee. At the same time, sink the left lower leg and foot. Simultaneously, guide the left lower arm and hand in front of the body following a clockwise arch until the palm of the hand faces the floor. The right hand approaches the head by releasing in the elbow.

2. Bend the right knee further. As you do so, place the left leg with the heel NE. Simultaneously, lower the left arm.

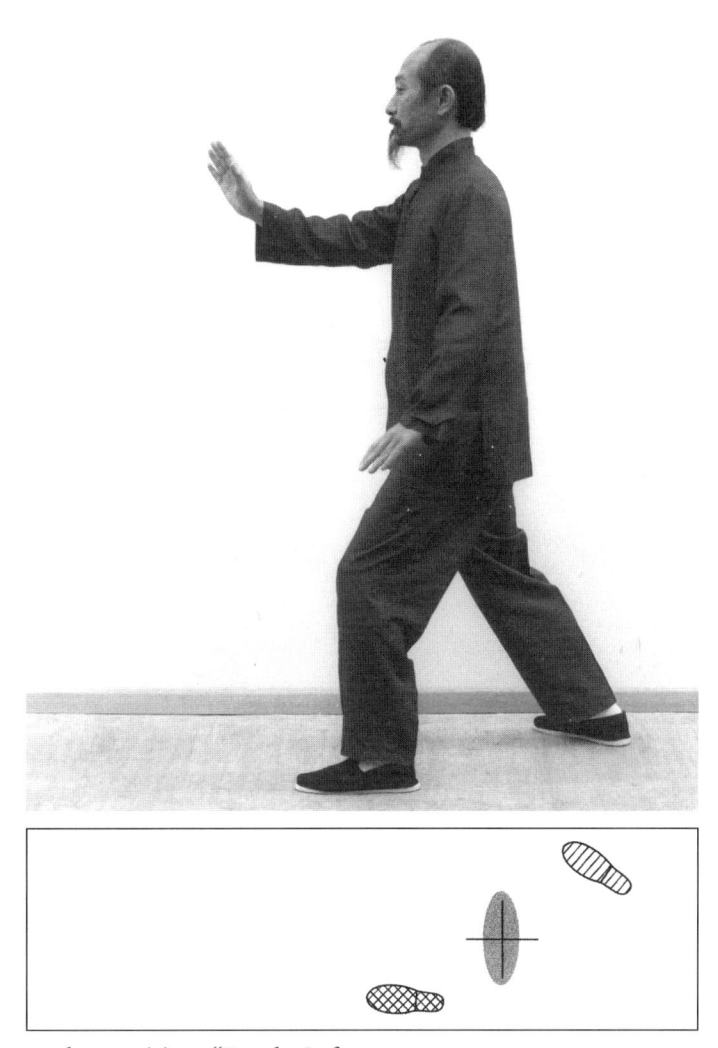

3. You repeat the position "Brush Left Knee—Twist Step" (see position 12, photo 3).

30. Brush Right Knee—Twist Step

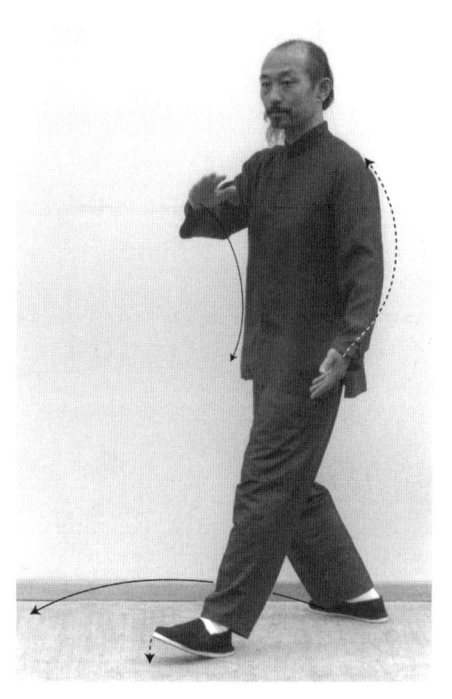

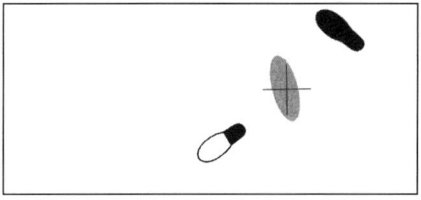

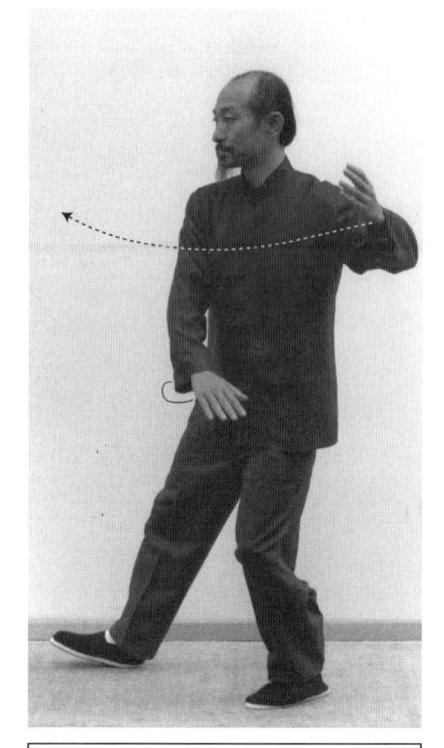

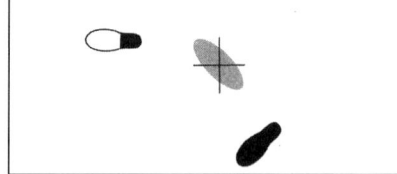

Not shown: Shift up to 90 percent of the weight onto the right foot. The positions of the arms remain the same.*

1. Turn the torso to the left until the front side faces NEE. At the same time, turn the left foot on the heel until the toes point NE. Simultaneously, turn the left hand slightly counterclockwise. Lower the right lower arm and hand in front of the body.†

*, † In their self-defense application, these movements happen simultaneously.

Not shown: Shift the weight onto the left foot. Sink the foot and bend the knee. While doing so, slightly lower the right arm in front of the body, the palm of the hand facing downward. Simultaneously, lift the left arm NNW to chest height.

2. Turn the torso somewhat to the left until the front side faces NE. At the same time, place the right leg forward (E) with the heel. Simultaneously, lower the right arm (hand at hip height). Lift the left arm to shoulder height and by bending the arm, guide the hand forward (hand at neck height).

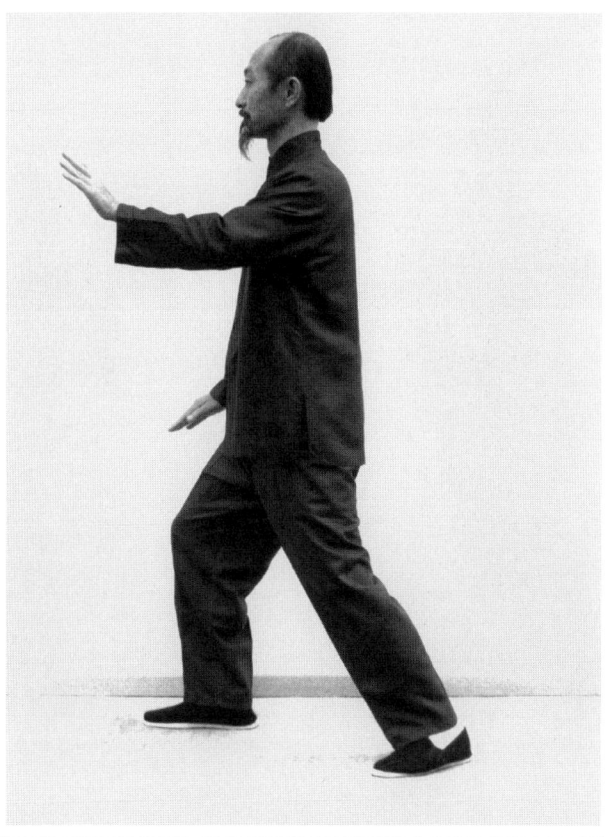

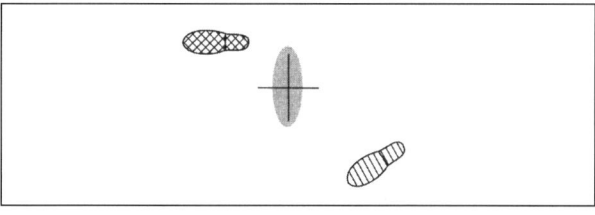

3. Turn the torso right until the front side faces E (Millstone Principle). At the same time, shift up to 70 percent of the weight onto the right foot, sink the foot and bend the knee. The arms follow the movement of the torso. Bring the left arm forward. Toward the end of this movement, slightly bend the hand (standing hand) and indicate a push. Guide the right arm in front of the body with the palm of the hand facing the body to the right side.

Finish by bending the hand slightly (standing hand).

The front right foot carries 70 percent of the weight and the back left foot 30 percent.

You are in the position "Brush Right Knee—Twist Step."

31. Step Forward and Strike with Fist

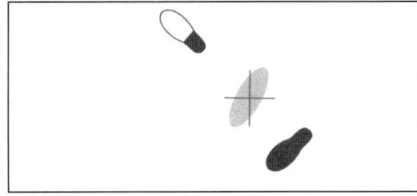

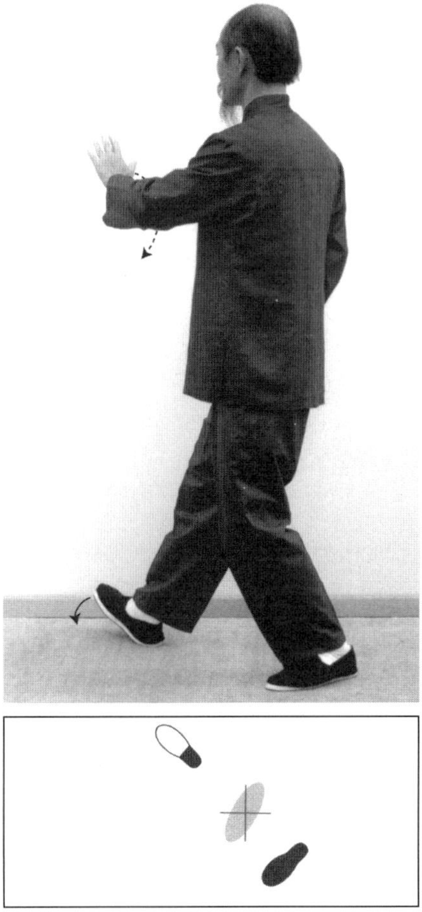

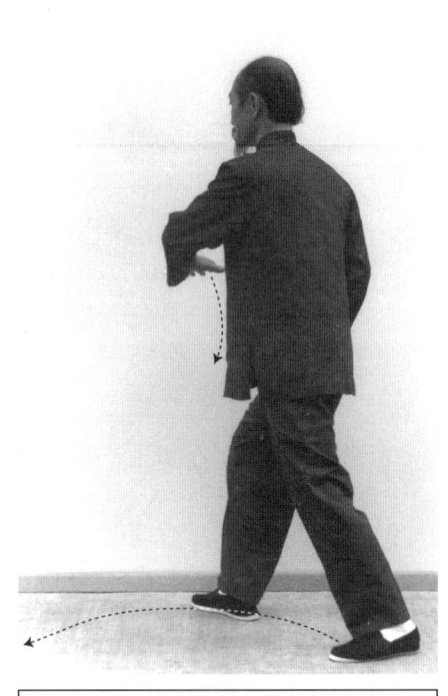

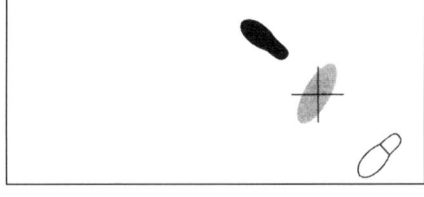

1. Turn the torso and right leg on the heel to the right until the front side of the torso faces SEE and the toes point SE. At the same time, shift up to 90 percent of the weight onto the left foot and bend the knee. Simultaneously, guide the right hand to the right hip, the palm of the hand facing the body. Slightly lower the left lower arm and hand in front of the body.

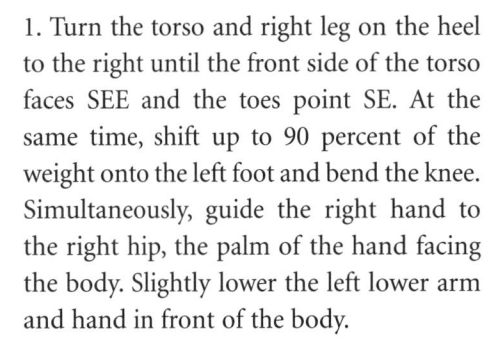

2. Shift up to 90 percent of your weight onto the right foot, sink the foot, and bend the knee. Simultaneously, slightly lower the left arm in front of the body with the palm of the hand facing downward.

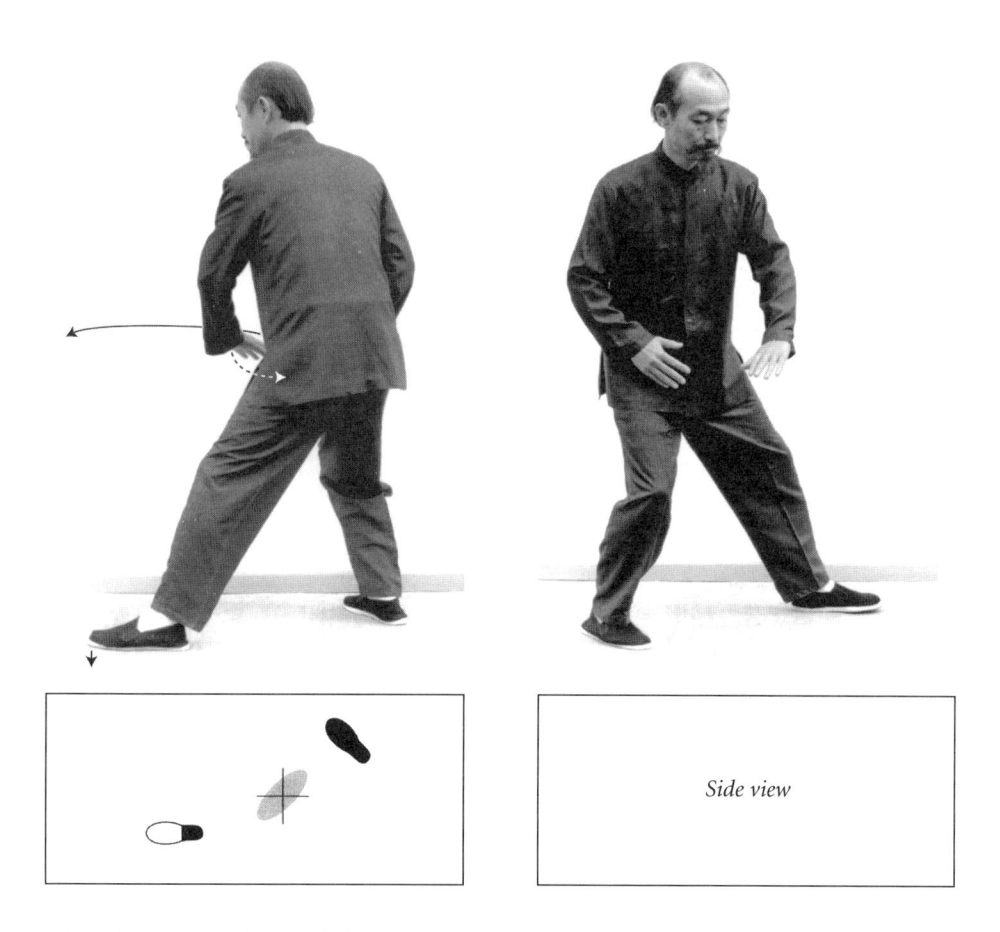

3. Turn the torso right until the front side faces SE. At the same time, place the left leg forward with the heel (E). Lower the left arm further in front of the body.

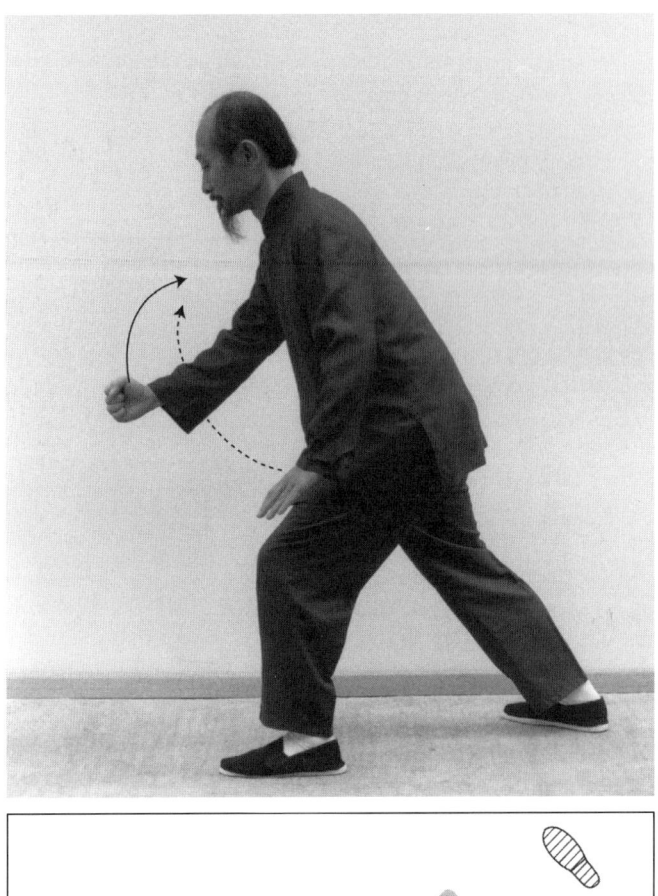

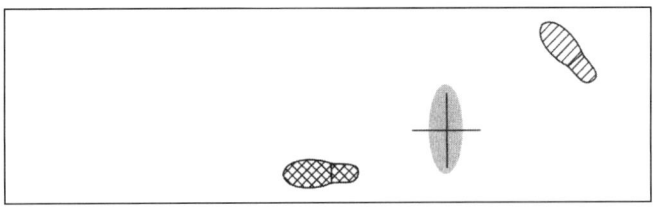

4. Turn the torso left until the front side faces E (Millstone Principle). At the same time, shift up to 70 percent of the weight onto the left foot, sink the foot, and bend the knee. Simultaneously, guide the left arm, hand passing the knee, left to the side of the body. Toward the end of this movement, slightly bend the hand (standing hand). Guide the right arm straight forward at hip level, and close the hand into a fist at the same time. Lean forward while turning the torso and shifting the weight. 70 percent of the weight rests on the front left foot and 30 percent on the back right foot.

You are in the position "Step Forward and Strike with Fist."

Note: This movement is easier to perform if one takes a Bow Step that is somewhat longer than usual.

Repetition

Ward-Off, Right (4)

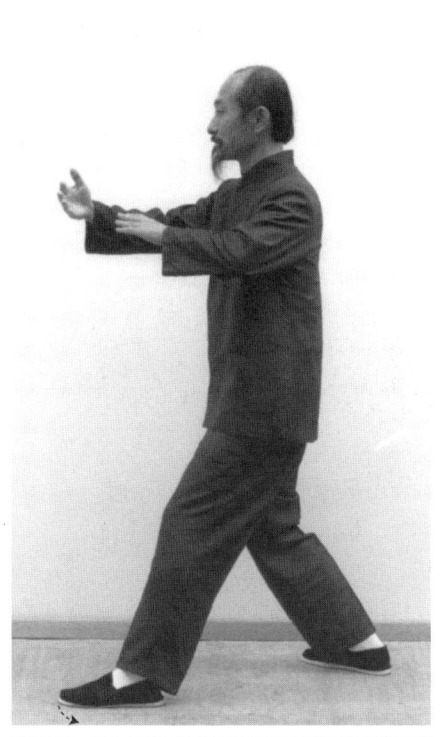

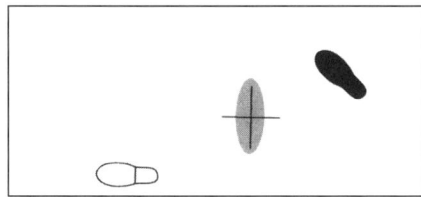

1. Shift up to 90 percent of the weight onto the back right foot. Bend the knee and straighten the torso. Simultaneously, lift both arms in front of the body and bring them together as in "Ward-Off, Right." At the same time, open the fist.

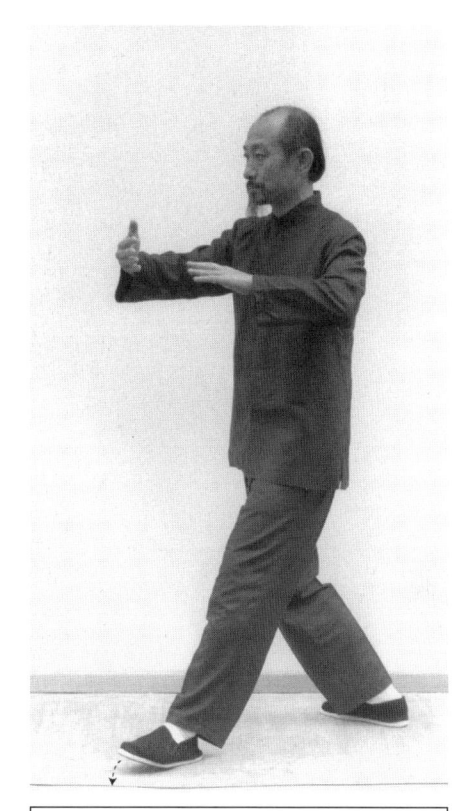

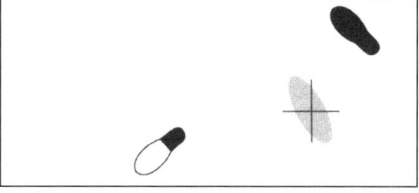

2. Turn the torso left until the front side faces NEE. At the same time, turn the left leg on the heel until the toes face NE. The arms maintain their positions as they follow the torso turn.

3. Not shown: Shift up to 90 percent of the weight onto the left foot, sink the foot, and bend the knee. The positions of the arms remain the same.

4. Not shown: Place the right leg forward (E) with the heel.

A repetition of these positions follows:

Rollback (5)

Press (6)

Push (7)

Single Whip (8)

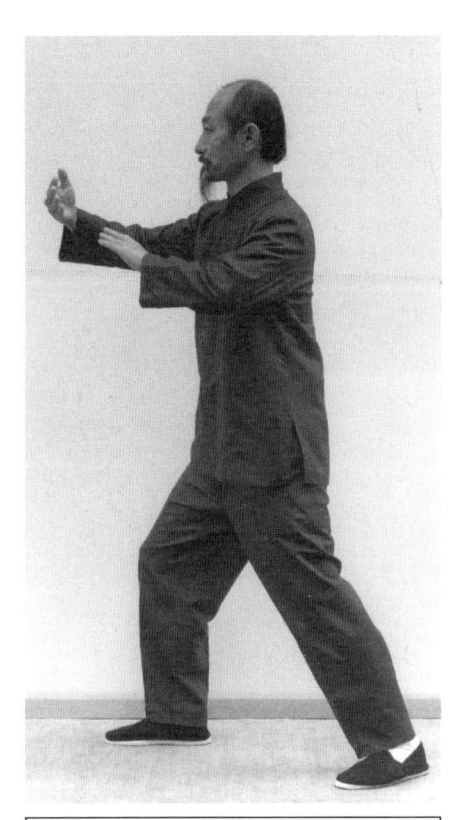

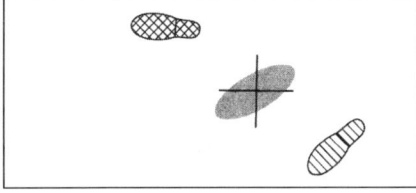

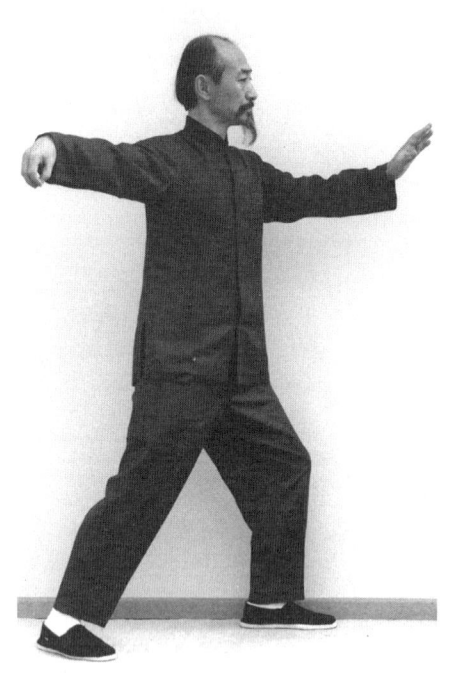

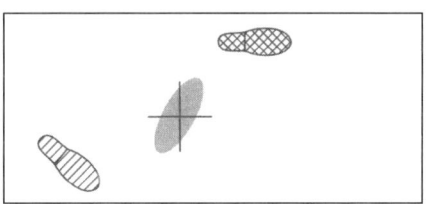

5. You repeat the position "Ward-Off, Right."

You are in the position "Single Whip."

Part 3

32. Fair Lady Works at Shuttle, Left

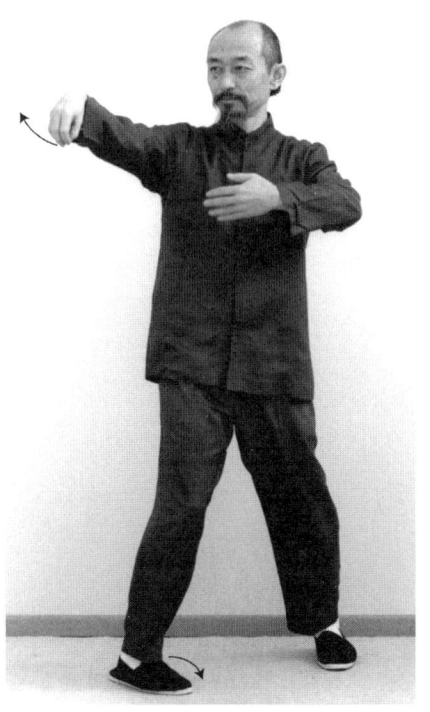

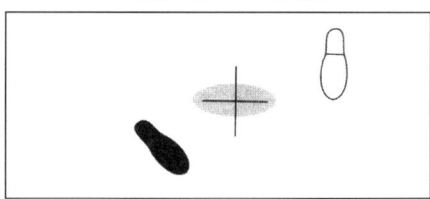

Not shown: Shift up to 90 percent of the weight onto the right foot and bend the knee. Sink the right arm somewhat by releasing in the elbow. Stretch the left arm somewhat forward until the palm of the hand faces the floor.

1. Turn the torso and left leg on the heel to the right until the front side of the torso and the toes face N. The left arm follows the movement of the torso. Guide the lower arm and hand as a unit in front of the body until the hand is in front of the breastbone (Ward-Off).

The palm of the hand faces the body. The position of the right arm remains the same. It faces NE.

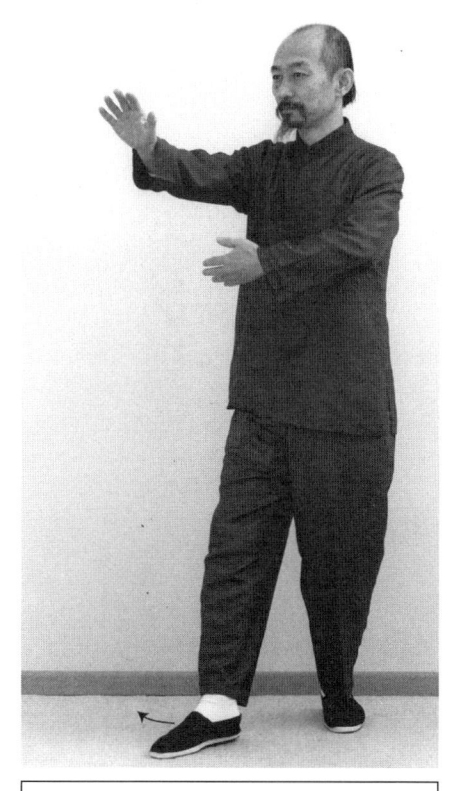

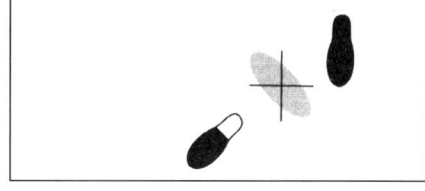

2. Turn the torso to the right until the front side faces NE. At the same time, shift up to 90 percent of the weight onto the left foot. The leg follows the movement of the torso with a lifted heel until the toes point NE. Simultaneously, slightly sink the right arm by releasing in the elbow and opening the "Bird's Head" upward. The left arm follows the movement of the torso.

3. Turn the torso to the right until the front side faces NEE. At the same time, place the right leg slightly forward (NE) with the heel. The toes point SEE. The arms follow the movement of the torso. Sink the left arm somewhat.

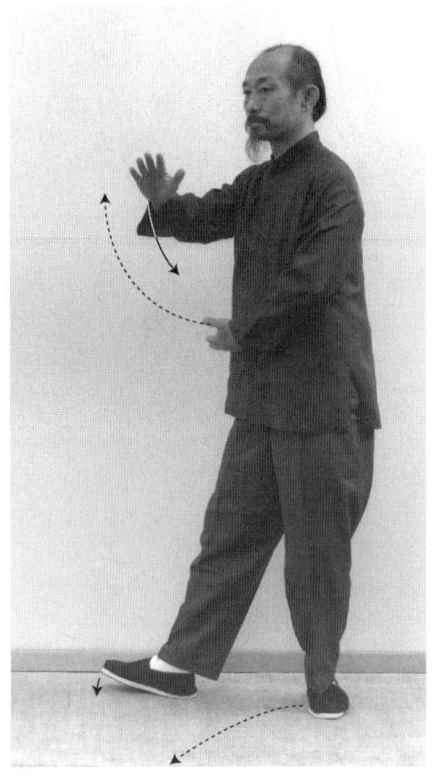

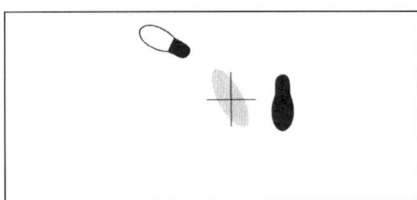

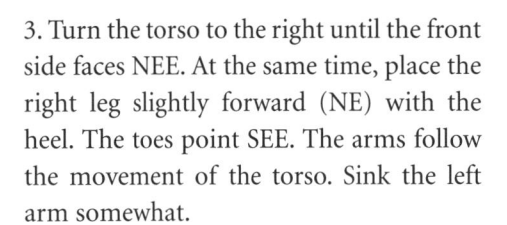

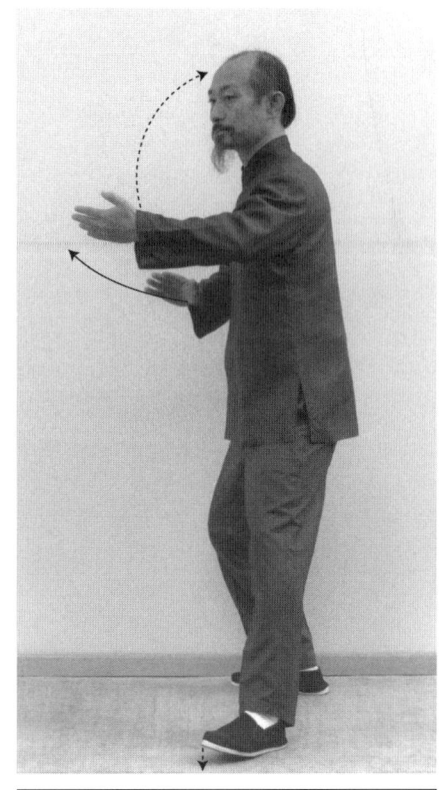

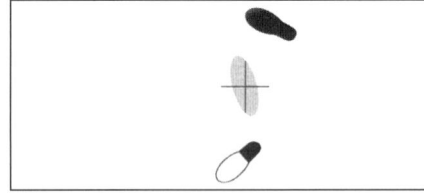

4. Turn the torso to the right until the front side faces E. While doing this, shift the weight completely onto the right foot, sink the foot, and bend the knee. As the weight shifts, place the left leg forward (NE) with the heel.

Simultaneously, lift the left arm forward and upward and lower the right arm in front of the body (palm of the hand facing downward). The position of the arms resembles "Ward-Off, Right" (reverse side).

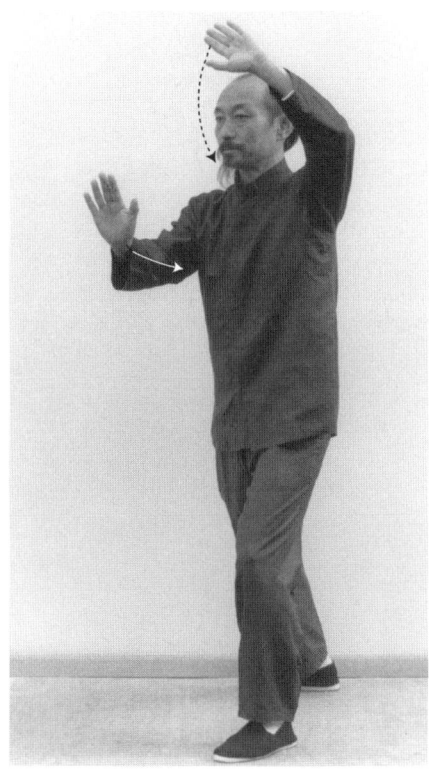

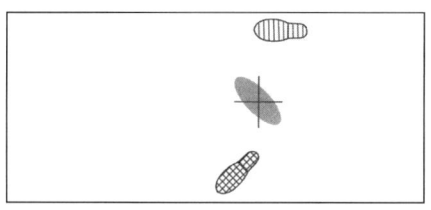

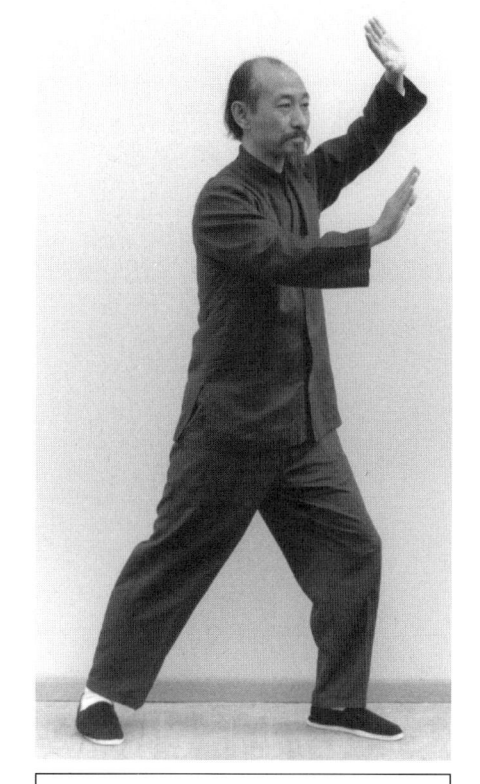

5. Turn the torso and right leg on the heel to the left until the front side of the torso faces NE and the toes point E (Millstone Principle, Bow Step). At the same time, shift up to 70 percent of the weight onto the front left foot, sink the foot, and bend the knee. The arms follow the movement of the torso. Lift the left arm in an arch forward and upward. At the same time, turn the lower arm and hand clockwise until the palm of the hand faces forward and upward.

Slightly lift the right arm in an arch and guide it forward (NE); the hand indicates a push. Toward the end of this movement, bend both hands slightly (standing hand).

70 percent of the weight rests on the front left foot and 30 percent on the back right foot.

You are in the position "Fair Lady Works at Shuttle, Left."

33. Fair Lady Works at Shuttle, Right

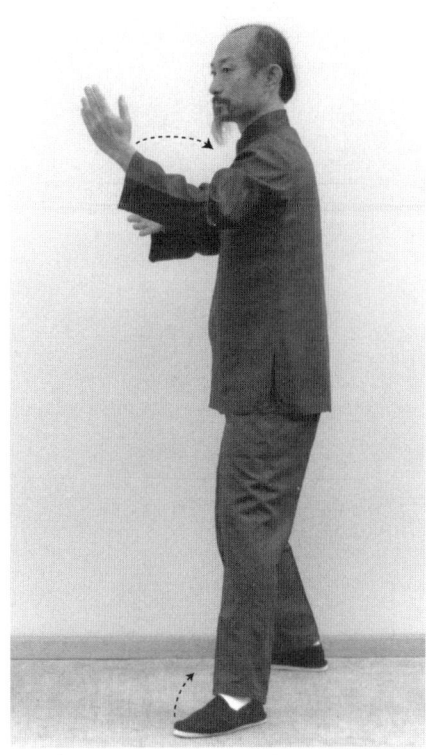

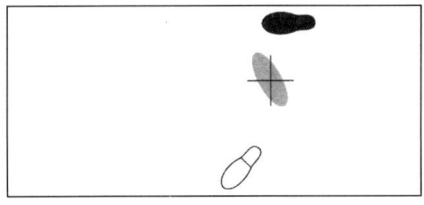

1. Turn the torso right until the front side faces NEE (Millstone Principle). At the same time, shift up to 90 percent of the weight onto the back right foot and bend the knee. Simultaneously, lower both arms and bring then together as in "Rollback" (reverse side!).

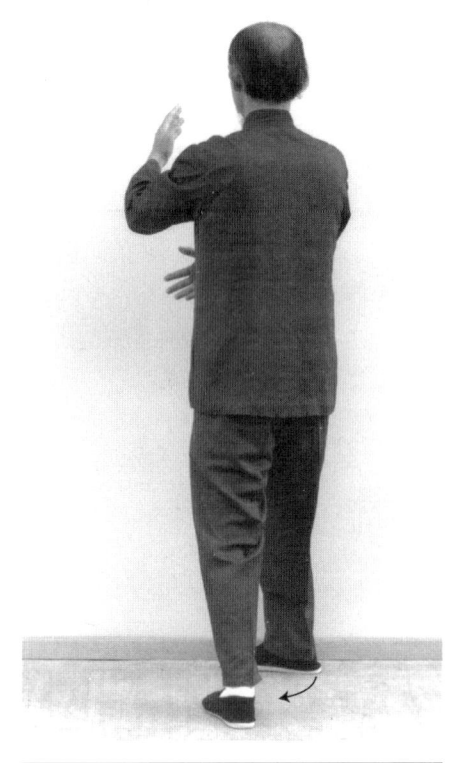

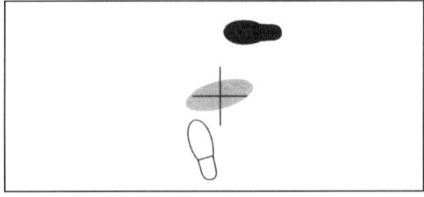

2. Turn the torso and left leg on the heel to the right until the front side of the torso and the toes point SSE. At the same time, guide the left lower arm and hand as one unit in front of the body until the hand is in front of the central axis. Lower the right arm slightly in front of the body. The left arm is above the right one, and both palms are turned to the body. (For the front view, see page 170.)

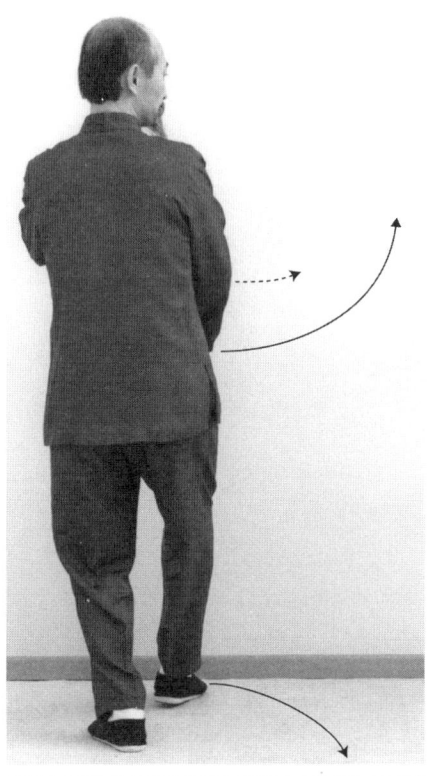

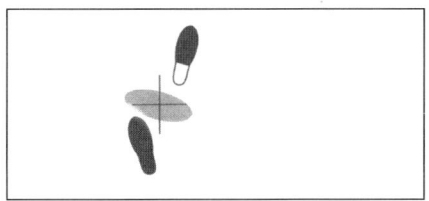

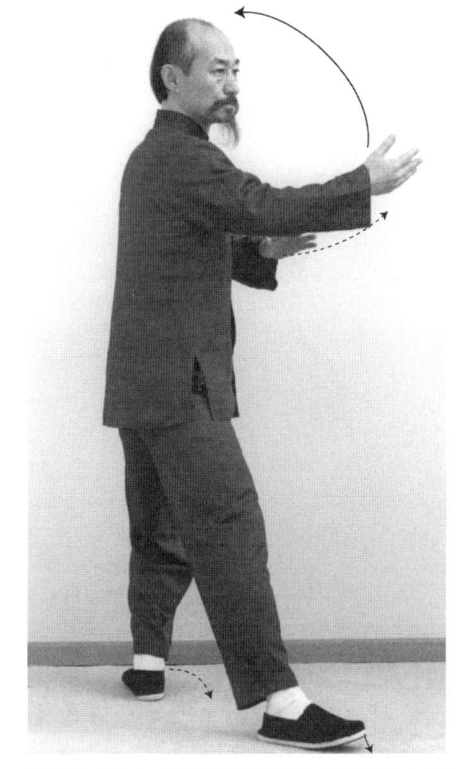

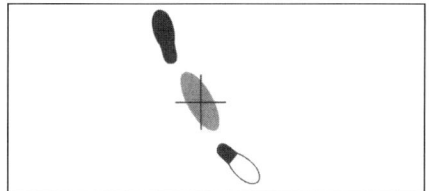

3. Turn the torso to the right until the front side faces SSW. At the same time, shift up to 90 percent of the weight onto the left foot and bend the knee. The right leg, heel raised, follows the movement of the torso until the toes point SSW.* Simultaneously, lower both arms slightly in front of the body. At the same time, turn the left palm somewhat downward and the right palm somewhat upward. (For the front view, see page 171.)

4. Turn the torso to the right until the front side faces W. As the torso turns, place the right leg with the heel NW. Simultaneously, guide the right arm to the right until it faces NW, the palm of the hand facing upward. Lower the left arm in front of the body. Turn the lower arm and hand clockwise until the palm of the hand faces downward. The position of the arms resembles "Ward-Off, Right."

*The turn can also be on the heel.

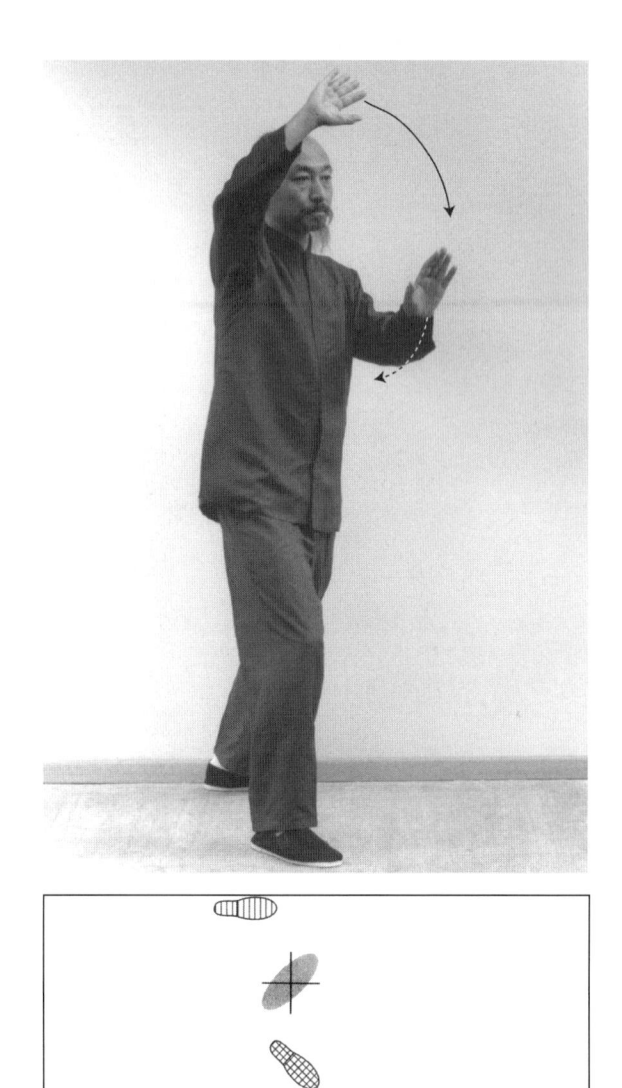

5. Turn the torso and left leg on the heel to the right until the front side of the torso faces NW and the toes point W (Millstone Principle, Bow Step). At the same time, shift up to 70 percent of the weight onto the right foot, sink the foot, and bend the knee. The arms follow the movement of the torso. Lift the right arm in an arch forward and upward. At the same time, turn the lower arm and hand counterclockwise until the palm of the hand faces forward and upward. Slightly lift the left arm in an arch and guide it forward (NW); the hand indicates a push. Toward the end of this movement, bend both hands slightly (standing hand).

70 percent of the weight rests on the front right foot and 30 percent on the back left foot.

You are in the position "Fair Lady Works at Shuttle, Right."

Repetition

Fair Lady Works at Shuttle, Left (32)

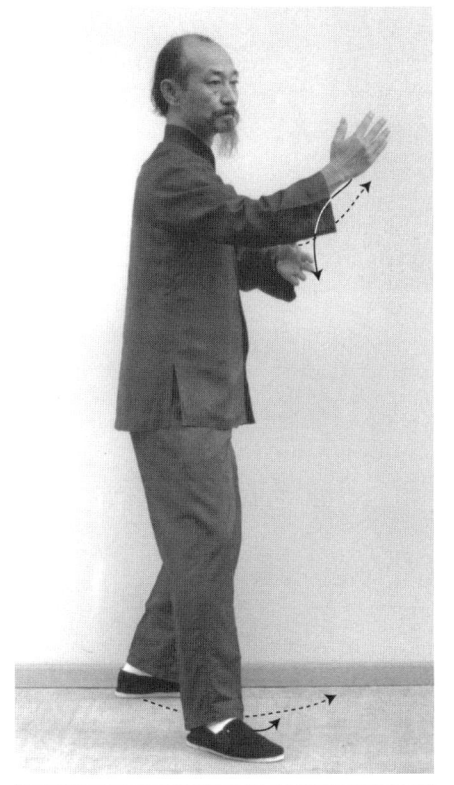

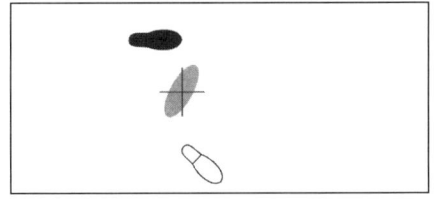

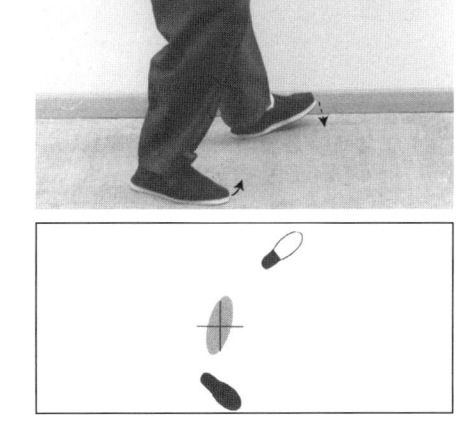

1. Turn the torso to the left until the front side faces NWW (Millstone Principle). At the same time, shift up to 90 percent of the weight onto the back left foot and bend the knee. Simultaneously, lower both arms and bring them together, as in "Rollback."

Not shown: Place the right leg a foot-length to the left. Place the heel first. The toes point NW.

2. Turn the torso to the left until the front side faces W. At the same time, shift the weight completely onto the right foot. During the torso turn and weight shift, place the left leg with the heel SW. Simultaneously, lift the left arm SW, palm of the hand facing upward. Lower the right arm, palm of the hand facing downward.

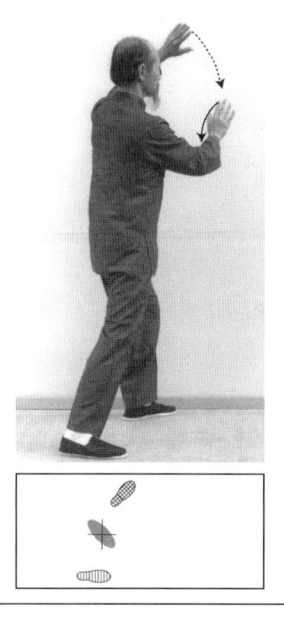

3. Turn the torso and the right leg on the heel to the left until the front side of the torso faces SW and the toes point W (Millstone Principle, Bow Step). At the same time, shift up to 70 percent of the weight onto the front left foot, sink the foot and bend the knee. Lift the arms forward and upward as described above.

You are in the position "Fair Lady Works at Shuttle, Left."

Fair Lady Works at Shuttle, Right (33)

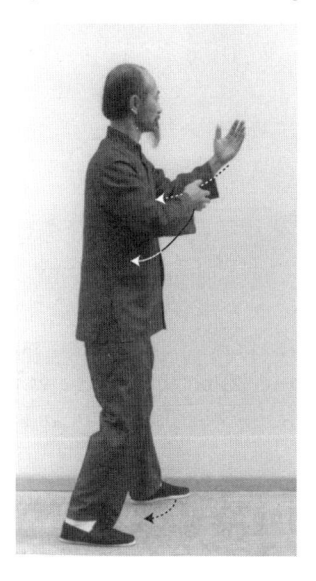

1. Turn the torso right until the front side faces SWW (Millstone Principle). At the same time, shift up to 90 percent of the weight onto the back right foot and bend the knee. Simultaneously, lower both arms and bring them together, as in "Rollback" (reverse side).

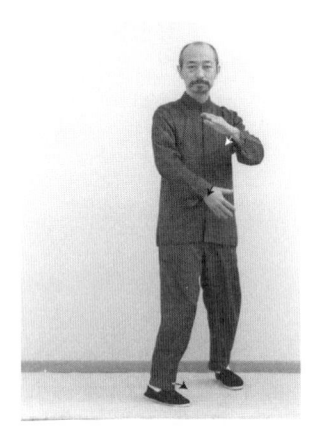

2. Turn the torso and left leg on the heel to the right until the front side of the torso and the toes are directed NNW. Simultaneously, guide the left lower arm and hand (as one unit) in front of the body until the hand is in front of the central axis. Lower the right arm slightly in front of the body. The left arm is over the right one. Both palms of the hands are turned toward the body.

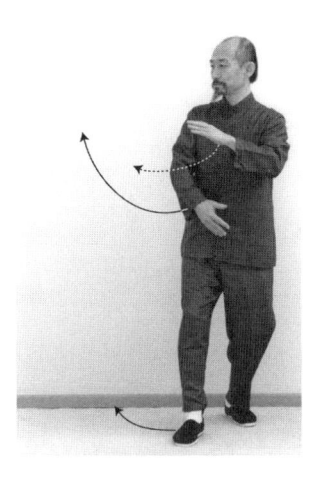

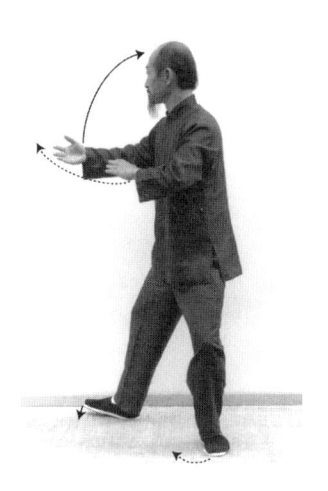

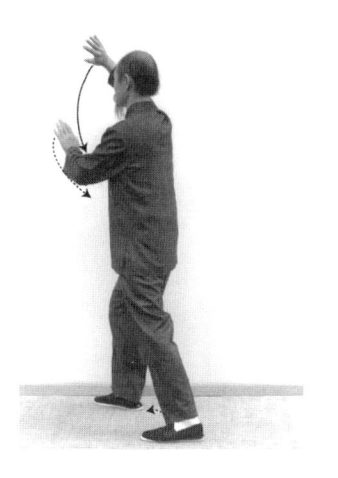

3. Turn the torso to the right until the front side faces NNE. At the same time, shift up to 90 percent of the weight onto the left foot and bend the knee. The right leg follows the movement of the torso with a raised heel until the toes point NNE.* Simultaneously, lower both arms slightly in front of the body. At the same time, turn the left palm somewhat downward and the right palm somewhat upward.

4. Turn the torso to the right until the front side faces E. At the same time, place the right leg with the heel SE. Simultaneously, guide the right arm to the right until it faces SE with the palm of the hand facing upward. Lower the left arm in front of the body; turn the lower arm and hand clockwise until the palm of the hand faces downward. The position of the arm resembles that of "Ward-Off, Right."

5. Turn the torso and the left leg on the heel until the front side of the torso faces SE and the toes point E (Millstone Principle, Bow Step). At the same time, shift up to 70 percent of the weight onto the right foot, sink the foot, and bend the knee.

The arms follow the movement of the torso, lifting them forward and upward as described above.

You are in the position "Fair Lady Works at Shuttle, Right."†

*The turn can also be on the heel.
†"Fair Lady Works at Shuttle" is used especially to counter Pa Kua attacks because its techniques use circular approaches.

Ward-Off, Left (3)

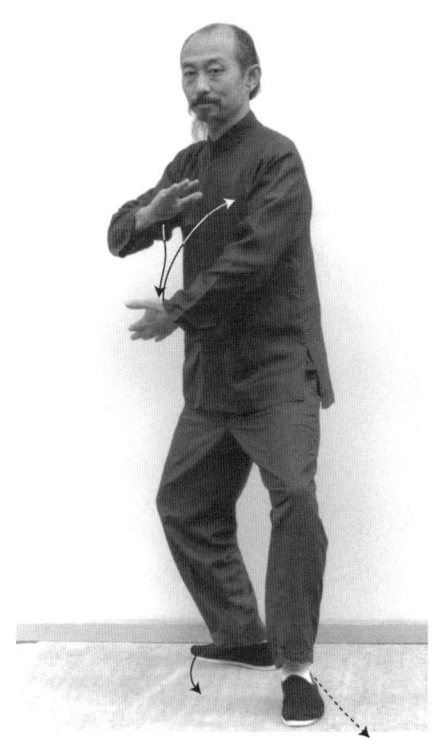

Ward-Off, Right (4)
Rollback (5)
Press (6)
Push (7)
Single Whip (8)

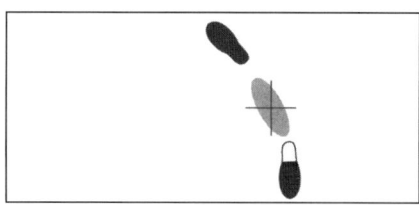

1. Turn the torso to the left until the front side faces NEE. At the same time, shift up to 90 percent of the weight onto the right foot and bend the knee (release in the right groin fold). The left leg follows the movement of the torso with a raised heel until the toes point N. Simultaneously, lower both arms in front of the body by releasing in the elbows and turn the palms to face each other.

Not shown: (a) Place the left leg to the left on the heel (NW).

(b) Turn the torso and right leg on the heel to the left until the front side of the torso faces N and the toes point NE (Millstone Principle, Bow Step). At the same time, shift up to 70 percent of the weight onto the front left foot. Simultaneously, raise the left arm and lower the right arm.

You are in the position "Ward-Off, Left."

Squatting Single Whip (24)

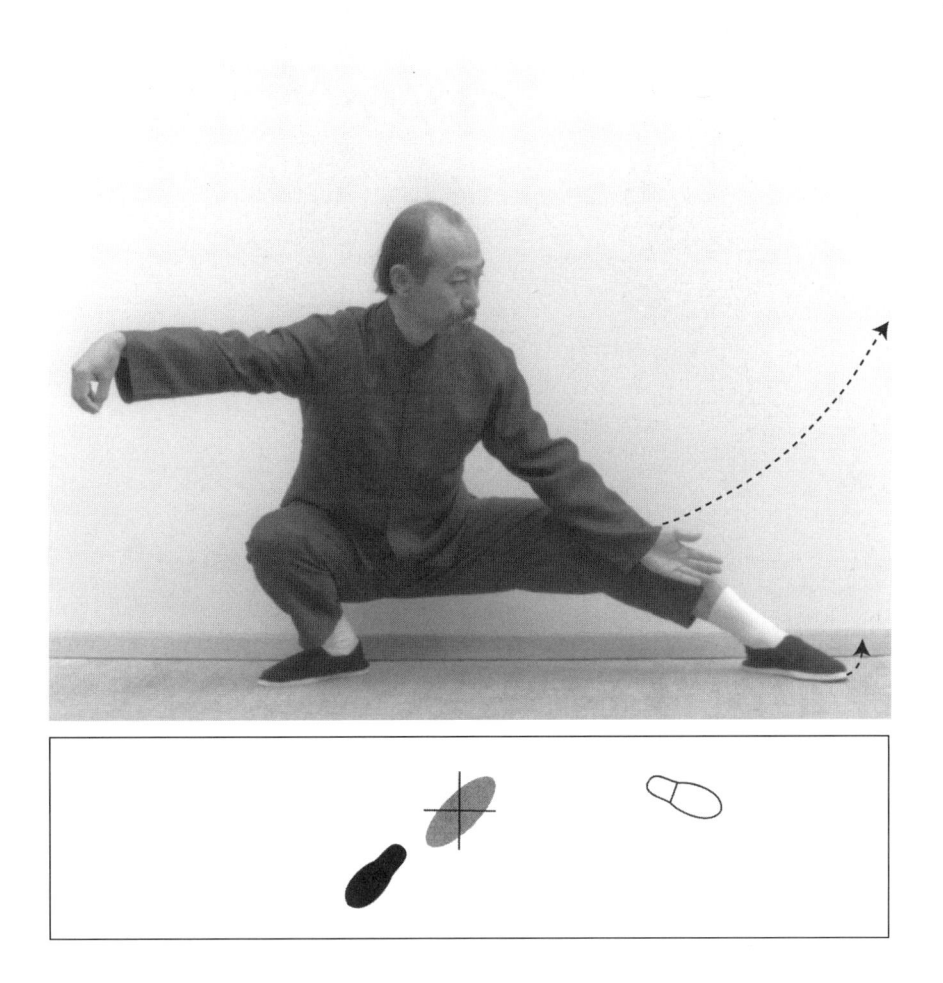

You are in the position "Squatting Single Whip."

34. Step Forward to Seven Stars

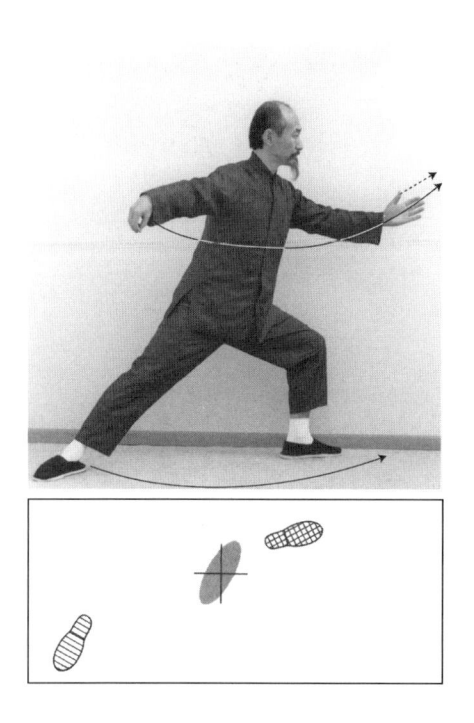

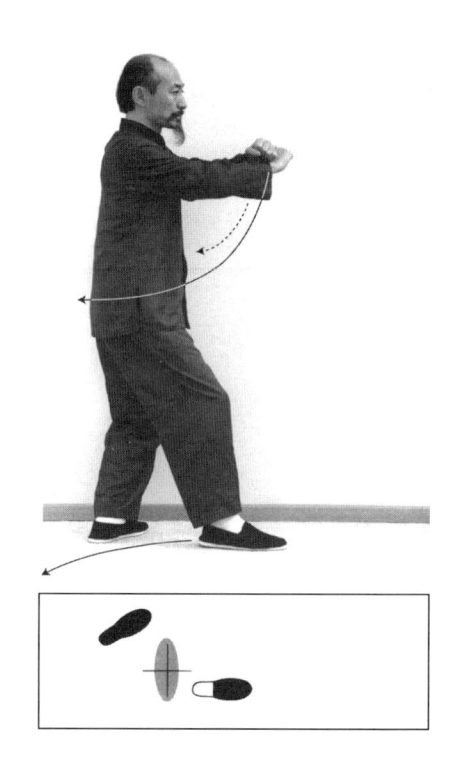

1. Turn the torso to the left until the front side faces NWW. At the same time, shift up to 70 percent of the weight onto the front left foot. As the torso turns, turn the left foot to the left without raising it. The toes point 30° away form direct W. Simultaneously, lift the left arm following an arch forward and upward until it is somewhat lower than the right arm.

2. Turn the torso to the left until the front side faces W. At the same time, shift the weight completely onto the left foot. Place the right leg forward (W) with the front part of the foot following an arch (Step of the Fishing Horse). Simultaneously, lift the left arm forward and upward in an arch that is directed slightly inward. Similarly, guide the right arm inward, forward, and upward. At the same time, first turn the hand clockwise and then open the "bird's head." Toward the end of this movement, bring the arms together in front of the breastbone with the wrists crossed and the hands closed into fists. The right arm is below the left one.

90 percent of the weight rests on the back left foot and 10 percent on the front right foot.

You are in the position "Step Forward to Seven Stars."

35. Step Back and Ride Tiger

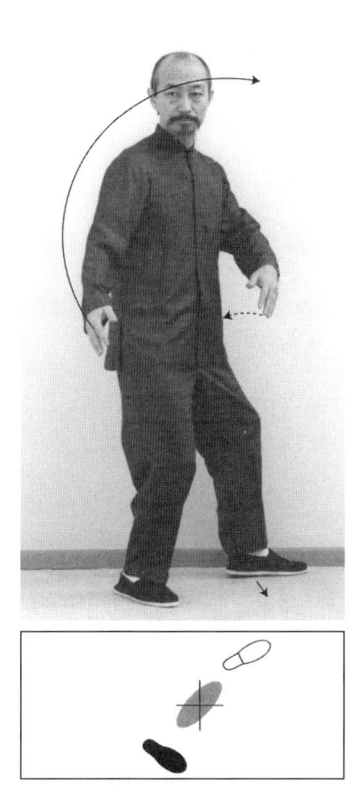

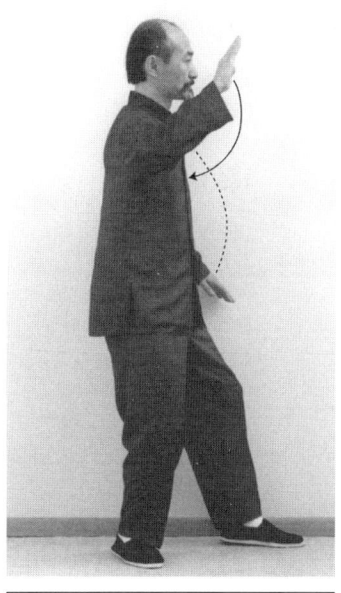

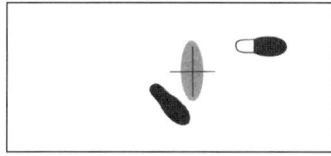

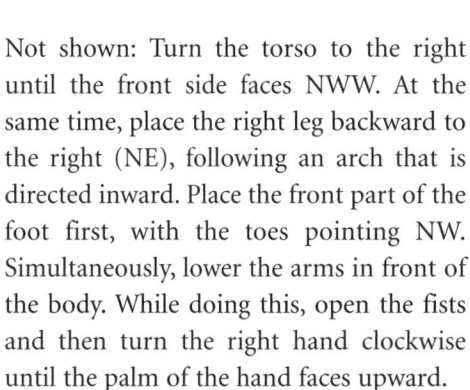

Not shown: Turn the torso to the right until the front side faces NWW. At the same time, place the right leg backward to the right (NE), following an arch that is directed inward. Place the front part of the foot first, with the toes pointing NW. Simultaneously, lower the arms in front of the body. While doing this, open the fists and then turn the right hand clockwise until the palm of the hand faces upward.

1. Turn the torso further to the right until the front side faces NW. At the same time, shift up to 90 percent of the weight onto the right foot and bend the knee. Simultaneously, continue to lower the arms and separate them.

2. Turn the torso to the left until the front side faces W. At the same time, shift the weight completely onto the right foot. As the torso turns, place the left leg somewhat to the right, setting down the front part of the foot first (Step of the Fishing Horse). The arms follow the movement of the torso. Lift the right arm following an arch at the side of your body, and then guide it forward and upward. Guide the left arm to the left side of the body. Toward the end of this movement, bend both hands somewhat (standing hand).

The back right foot carries 90 percent of the weight and the front left foot 10 percent.

You are in the position "Step Back and Ride Tiger."

36. Turn and Sweep over Lotus with Leg

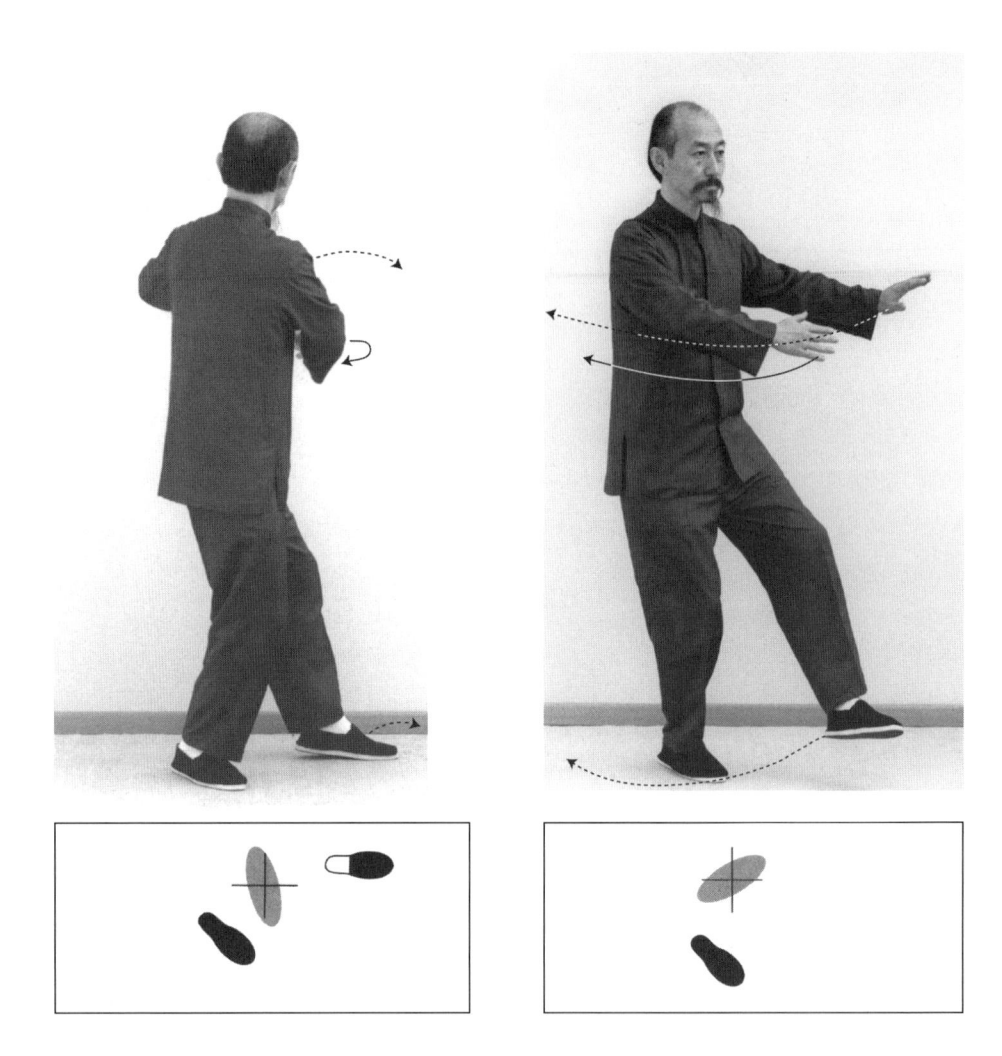

1. Turn the torso to the left until the front side faces SWW. At the same time, lower the right arm to the left, the palm facing the body. Lift the left arm to the left at chest level while turning the lower arm and hand slightly counterclockwise.

(For the position of the arm, see the next photo.)

2. Turn the torso to the right until the front side faces NNW. The left leg and the arms follow the movement of the torso.

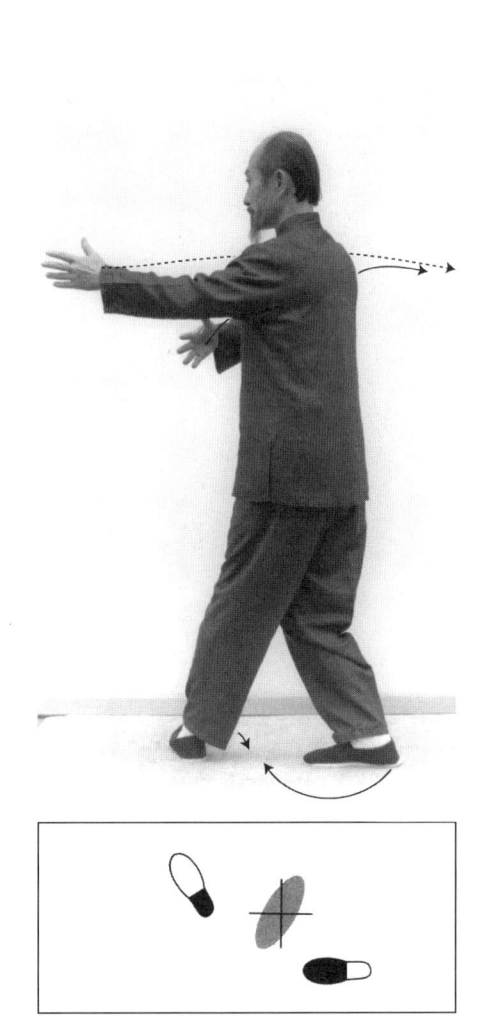

3. Turn the torso and right leg on the front part of the foot to the right until the front side faces SEE and the toes point E. Following the torso turn, place the left leg SEE, with the heel (toes point SSE). At the same time, shift up to 50 percent of your weight onto the left foot. The arms follow the movement of the torso.

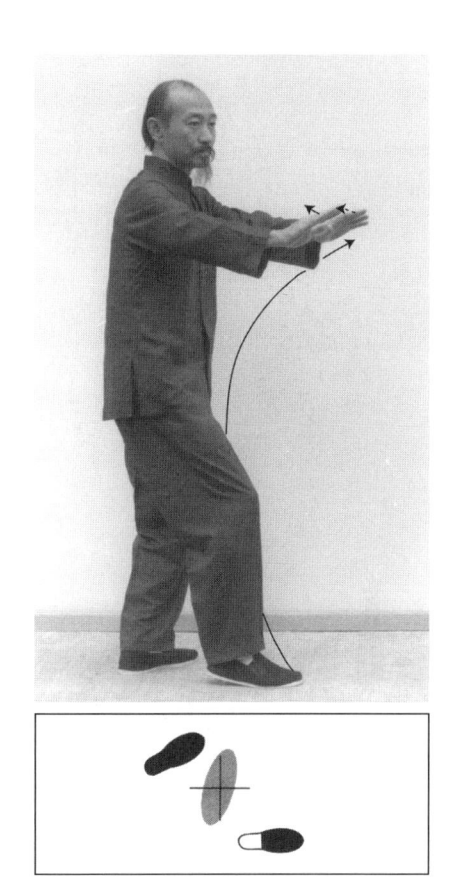

4. Turn the torso to the right until the front side faces W. Accompany the torso turn by turning the left foot further on the heel until the toes point 30° away from direct W. At the same time, shift up to 90 percent of the weight onto the left foot. The right leg follows the movement of the torso with a raised heel until the toes point W (Step of the Fishing Horse). The arms follow the movement of the torso. Lift the right arm while turning the lower arm and hand counterclockwise until the palm of the hand faces downward. Turn the left lower arm and hand somewhat clockwise until the palm of the hand faces to the floor. Toward the end of the movement, guide both arms slightly to the right while maintaining their parallel position.

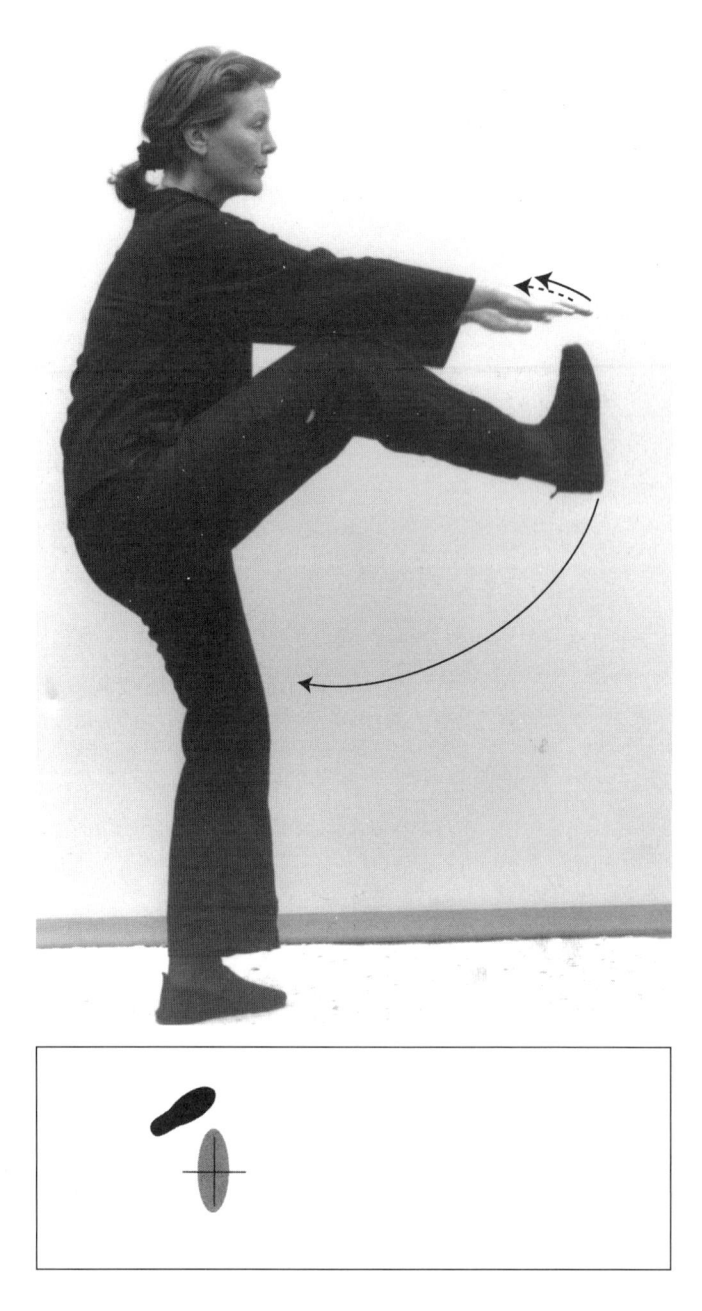

5. Turn the torso somewhat to the left and stretch the left leg slightly. At the same time, lift the right leg following an arch to the left. Then turn the torso somewhat to the right and guide the leg to the right in an arch, the toes pointing upward. Simultaneously, guide the arms somewhat to the left.

The front side of the torso faces W.

The weight rests on the left foot.

You are in the position "Turn and Sweep over Lotus with Leg."

37. Bend Bow and Shoot Tiger

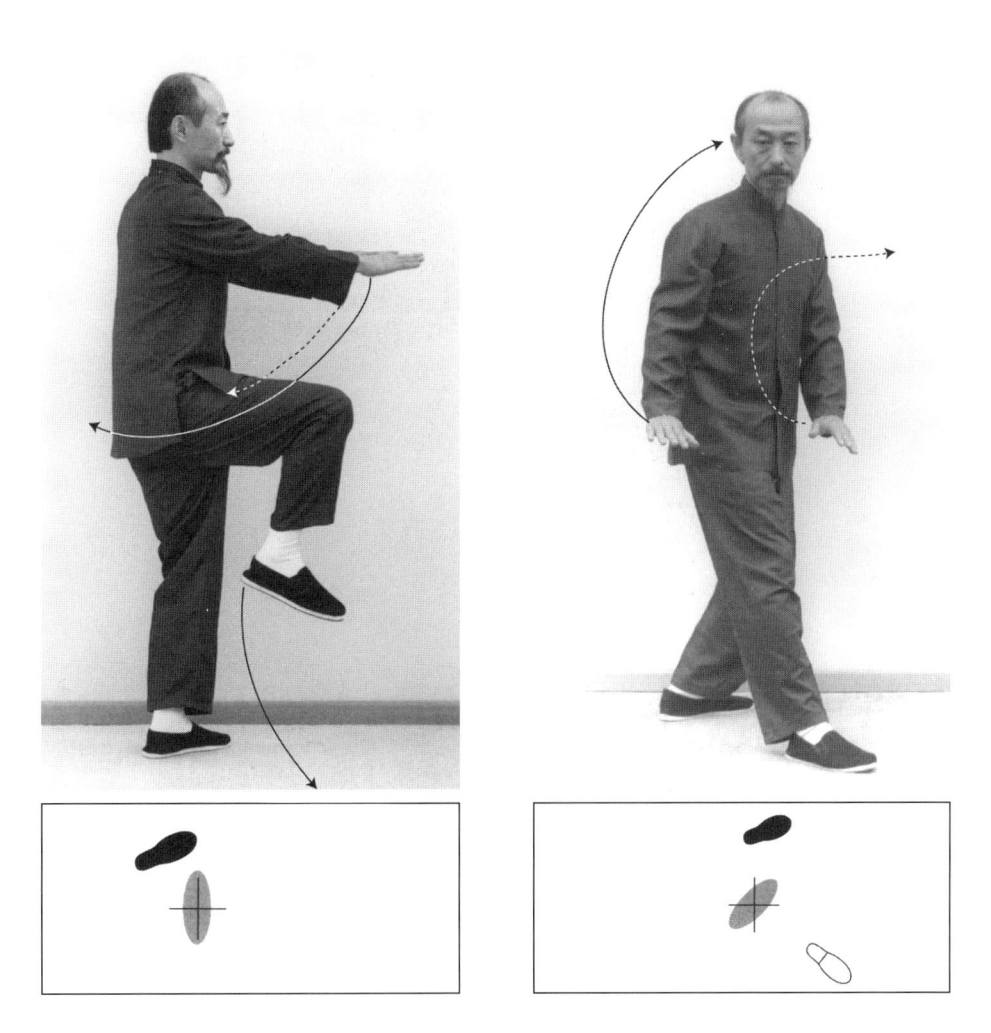

1. Sink the right lower leg (calf) and foot. Simultaneously, guide the arms farther left until the fingertips face SWW.

2. Turn the torso to the right until the front side faces NWW. At the same time, place the right leg with the heel first NW; the toes point NW. Simultaneously, lower the arms in their parallel position following a large arch and guide them to the right.

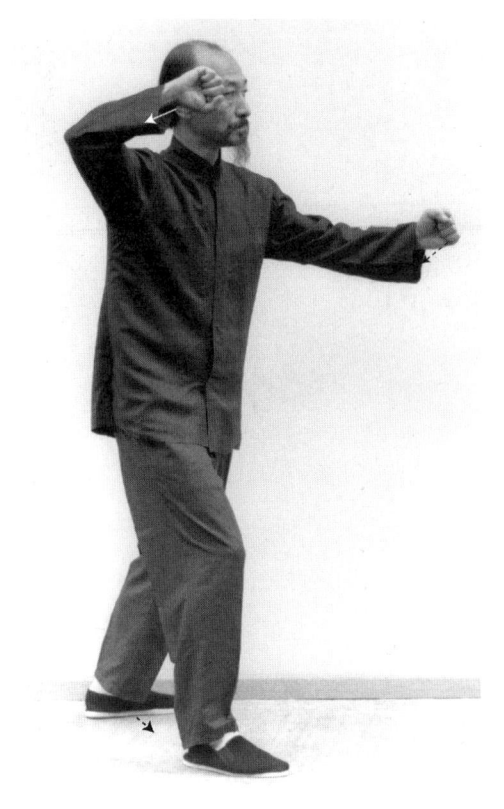

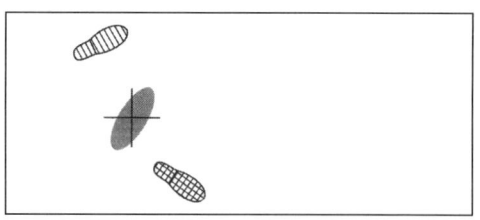

3. a) Turn the torso to the right until the front side faces NW. At the same time, shift up to 30 percent of the weight onto the right leg. The arms follow the torso turn to the right in their parallel position.

b) Turn the torso to the left until the front side faces NWW (Millstone Principle). At the same time, shift up to 70 percent of the weight onto the front right foot and bend the knee. Simultaneously, guide the arms forward and upward following arches (W).

Toward the end of the movement, close the hands into fists.

The front side of the torso faces NWW. You look W.

70 percent of the weight rests on the front right foot and 30 percent on the back left foot.

You are in the position "Bend Bow and Shoot Tiger."

Repetition

Step Forward, Deflect Downward, Parry, and Punch (14)

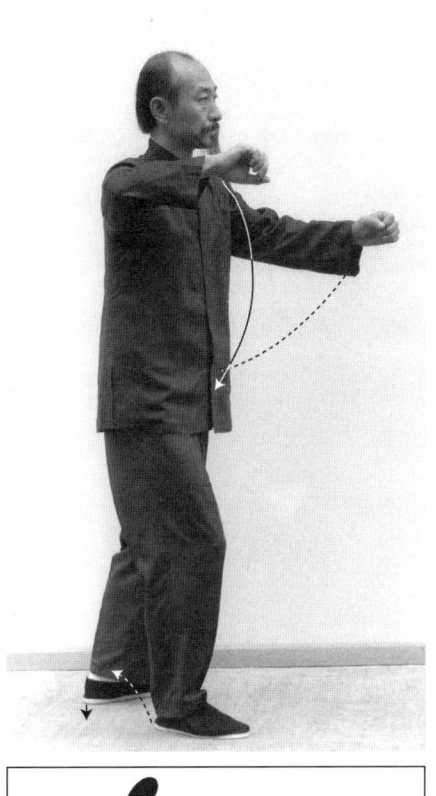

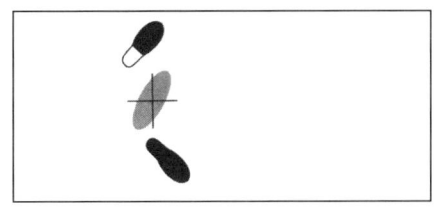

1. By releasing in the right groin fold, shift the weight completely onto the right foot and bend the knee. At the same time, place the left leg with the front of the foot at a distance of a foot length to the NW; the toes point SW. Simultaneously, lower the arms somewhat and open the fists.

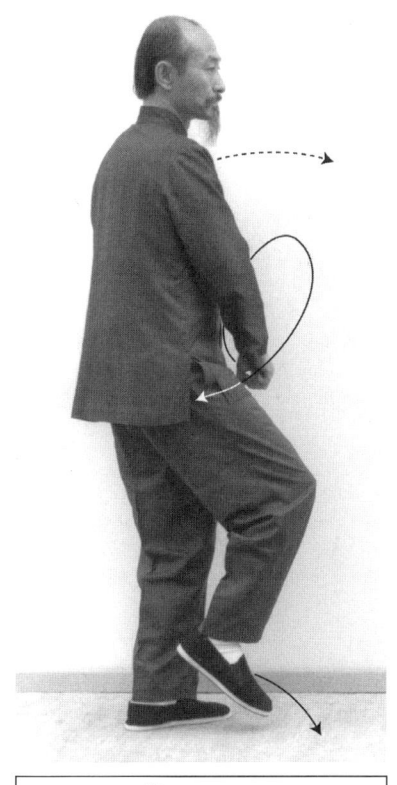

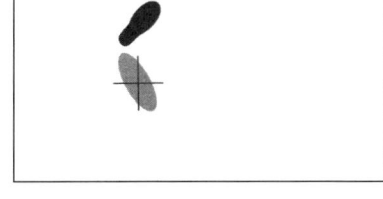

2. While shifting the weight completely onto the left foot, turn the torso to the left until the front side faces SWW. Pull the right leg to the left. The arms follow the movement of the torso. Lower them first in front of the body following an arch. Then continue to move them to the left side of the body. When lowering the arms, open the fists entirely and then close the right hand into a fist again.

You repeat the position "Parry and Punch" (see position 14, photos 4–6).

Withdraw and Push (15)

Cross Hands (16)

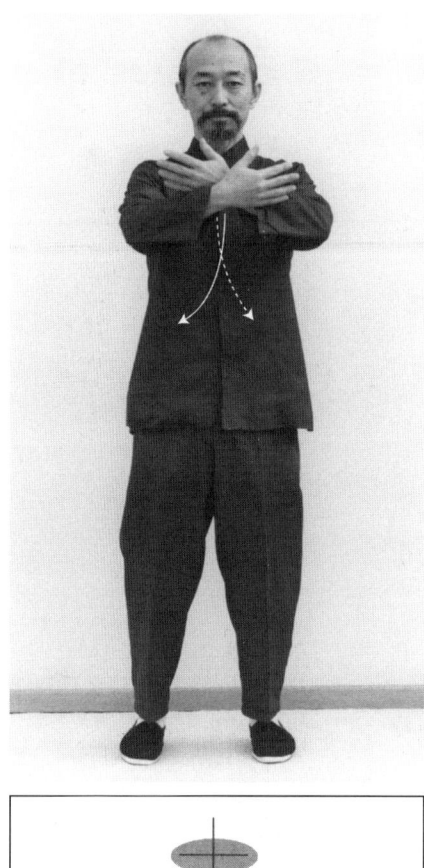

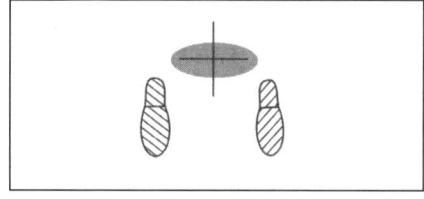

You are in the position "Cross Hands."

The weight is evenly distributed on both feet.

Conclusion

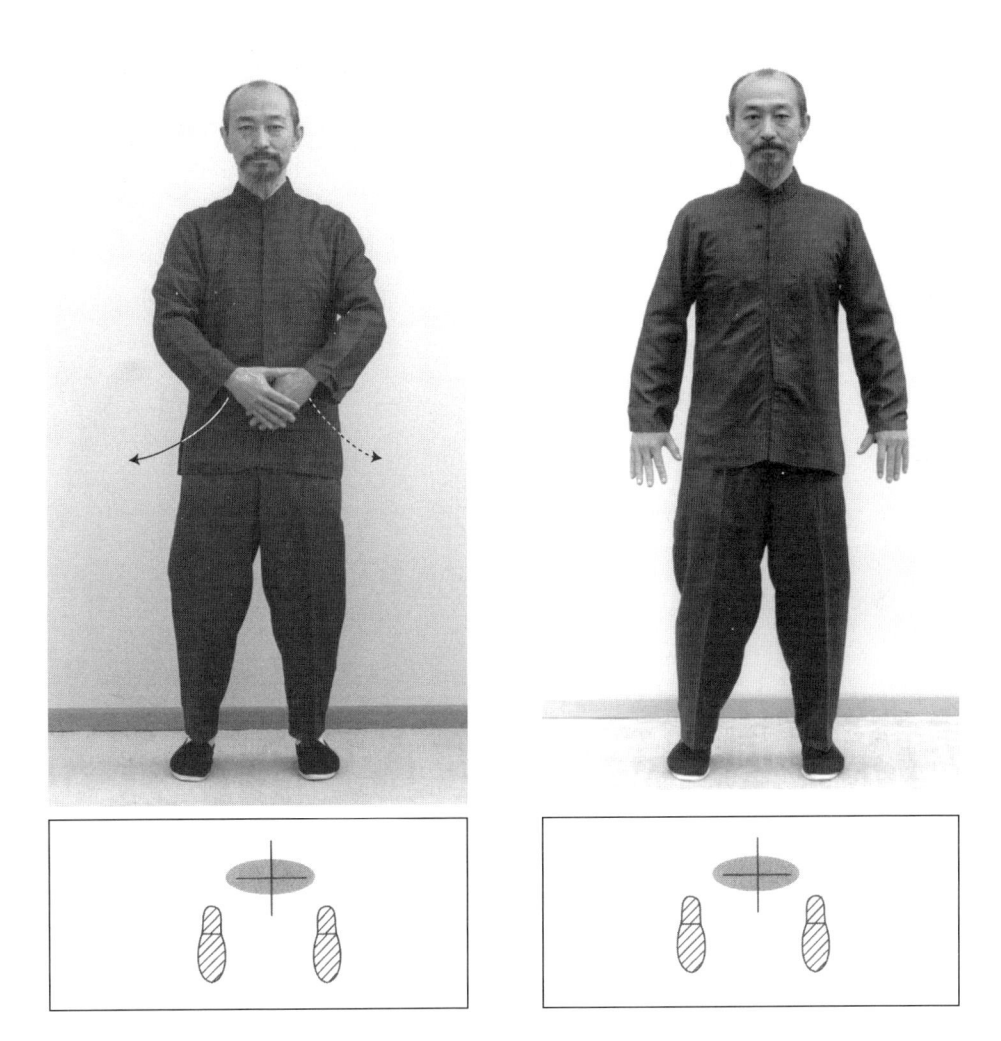

1–2: Slowly straighten the legs. Simultaneously, lower the arms. Then gradually move the arms apart and lower them to the sides of the body. Toward the end of this movement, slightly bend the hands (standing hand).

GLOSSARY

Chang San-Feng
Taoist master (end of the Sung Dynasty, 1127–1279), founder of T'ai Chi Ch'uan from the Yang-style point of view; known from the legends as a man of unusually large body size.

Ch'i
Cosmic or inner energy (Japanese: Ki; Indian: Prana).

Chi Chiang Tao (1920–1994)
Dr. Chi Chiang Tao was born in northern China in 1920. In 1937, he began his study of T'ai Chi Ch'uan because of a serious illness. He first learned the old Yang Pan Hou–style from Tien Cheng-Feng, among others. In 1948, he went to Taiwan and became a student of Cheng Man-Ch'ing. Today, he is still remembered as one of the best-known T'ai Chi masters in Taiwan and was a member of the Taiwan T'ai Chi Association, a union of students in the Cheng Man-Ch'ing tradition there. He was a master of T'ai Chi sword. In Taiwan, he practiced traditional Chinese medicine in addition to his teaching activities. In 1980, he moved to Vancouver, Canada.

Chi Kung
A collective term for mostly old Chinese health exercises specifically applied for individual problems that affect the activation of the Ch'i.

Chin
The special abilities that result from the development and use of the Ch'i that are understood to be separate energies; for example, Ting Chin (hearing energy), Tung Chin (interpreting energy), T'i Chin (uprooting energy).

Classical Treatises
Texts from the old masters in which the principles are written down. The most important ones are: Chang San Feng, *The Classical Text of T'ai Chi Ch'uan*; Wang Tsung Yueh, *The Theory of T'ai Chi Ch'uan*; and Wu Yu-Hsiang, *The Practice of the Basic 13 Positions*.

Hsing I Ch'uan
"Mind boxing," founder uncertain, either: Yueh Fei (tenth century) or Chi Ling-Feng (seventeenth century). Hsing I Ch'uan and Pa Kua belong to the "internal martial arts," as does T'ai Chi Ch'uan.

Kung Fu
Literally, "perfection" or "high technique." From time immemorial, the name Kung Fu has been used in China for martial arts that emphasize muscular force in order to express

their claim to the sheer perfection of their art. With time, Kung Fu has become the normal generic term for this type of martial art. Kung Fu, however, is still used in its original meaning. A perfection in any art is a "Kung Fu" in this art.

Pa Kua
The "Boxing of the Eight Diagrams," origin unknown; first known master was Tung Hai-Ch'uan (nineteenth century).

Push Hands (Tui Shou)
The most important partner exercise in Yang-style; based on the basic positions of Ward-Off, Rollback, Press, and Push.

Subtle Energy Realm
The entire subtle energy phenomena, such as the Ch'i, the meridian system, the subtle energy centers, aura, and so on.

T'ai Chi Ch'uan
Putting together "T'ai Chi" and "Ch'uan." "T'ai Chi" = the mother of Yin and Yang, synonymous with the Tao; Ch'uan = hand or fist. The name T'ai Chi Ch'uan results logically: through the hand or fist, in the method of the exercise, so to be attuned with the Tao.

Ta Lu
"The large rollback"; partner exercise.

Tan T'ien
Lower, middle, and upper Tan T'ien—the three Tan T'iens are the most important subtle energy centers in the Taoist tradition.

Tao
The Ultimate, Nameless, the Mother of the myriad things.

Tenacious Energy
Description of the accumulated Ch'i that has become "viscous."

Yang Lu-Ch'an
Founder of the Yang-style (1799–1872).

Yin and Yang
They represent all pairs of opposites. The alignment of T'ai Chi Ch'uan with the Yin and Yang demonstrates itself in the continuous changes in the movement from full to empty, weighted to unweighted, open to closed, and so on.

BIBLIOGRAPHY

Buber, Martin, comp. *Reden und Gleichnisse des Tschuang-Tse.* Frankfurt: Insel Taschenbuch, 1981. (Available in German only.)

Cheng Man-Ch'ing. *Advanced T'ai Chi Form Instructions.* Douglas Wile, comp. and trans. Brooklyn: Sweet Ch'i Press, 1985.

———. *Cheng Tzus's Thirteen Treatises on T'ai Chi Ch'uan.* Benjamin Pang Jeng Lo and Martin Inn, trans. Berkeley, CA: North Atlantic Books, 1985. (New translation from the original Chinese of the Thirteen Chapters on T'ai Chi Ch'uan.)

———. *Thirteen Chapters on T'ai Chi Ch'uan.* Douglas Wile, trans. Brooklyn: Sweet Ch'i Press, 1982.

Cheng Man-Ch'ing and Robert Smith. *T'ai Chi: The "Supreme Ultimate" Exercise for Health and Self-Defense.* Rutland, VT: Charles E. Tuttle Co., 1967.

Chen Wei-Ming. *T'ai Chi Ch'uan Ta Wen: Questions and Answers on T'ai Chi Ch'uan.* Berkeley, CA: North Atlantic Books, 1985.

Huang Wen-Shan. *Fundamentals of T'ai Chi Ch'uan.* Hong Kong: South Sky Book Company, 1973.

Jou Tsung Hwa. *The Dao of Taijiquan: Way to Rejuvenation.* Rutland, VT: Charles E. Tuttle Co., 1989.

Kobayashi, Petra. *Der Weg des T'ai Chi Ch'uan.* Munich: Hugendubel Verlag, 1984. (Available in German only.)

Kobayashi, Toyo and Petra. *T'ai Chi Ch'uan: Handbuch zum Selbststudium.* Munich: Hugendubel Verlag, 1979. (Available in German only.)

Matsuda. *History of the Chinese Martial Arts.* Tokyo: Shinjinbutsu Oraisha. (Available in Japanese only.)

———. *Secret of Chin Jia T'ai Chi.* Tokyo: Shinjinbutsu Oraisha. (Available in Japanese only.)

Wile, Douglas, trans. *Tai Chi Touchstones: Yang Family Secret Transmissions.* Brooklyn: Sweet Ch'i Press, 1983.

MORE BOOKS FROM THE TUTTLE MARTIAL ARTS LIBRARY

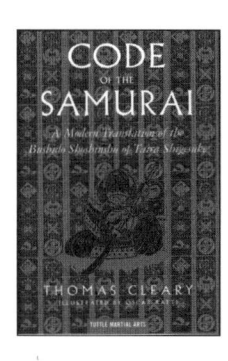

CODE OF THE SAMURAI
A Modern Translation of the Bushido Shoshinshu of Taira Shigesuke
by Thomas Cleary
5 X 7 ½, 128 pp., Hardcover, $14.95
ISBN-10: 0-8048-3190-4
ISBN-13: 978-0-8048-3190-1

A powerful contemporary translation of the classic treatise of the Way of the Warrior—still the core of Japanese social, political, and corporate structure—as compelling now as when it was first written 400 years ago.

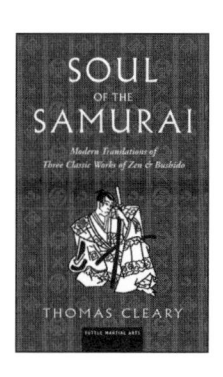

SOUL OF THE SAMURAI
Modern Translations of Three Classic Works of Zen and Bushido
by Thomas Cleary
5 X 7 ½, 160 pp., Hardcover, $14.95
ISBN-10: 0-8048-3690-6
ISBN-13: 978-0-8048-3690-6

This modern translation of three classics of martial arts philosophy reveals the powerful influence of Zen—and captures the true soul of the samurai.

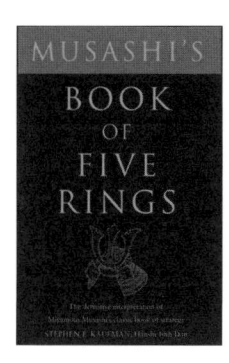

MUSASHI'S BOOK OF FIVE RINGS
The Definitive Interpretation of Miyamoto Musashi's Classic Book of Strategy
by Stephen F. Kaufman
5 ½ X 8 ½, 128 pp., Paperback, $13.95
ISBN-10: 0-8048-3520-9
ISBN-13: 978-0-8048-3520-6

A definitive treatise on mortal combat from one of Japan's most formidable warriors—the martial arts luminary Miyamoto Musashi.

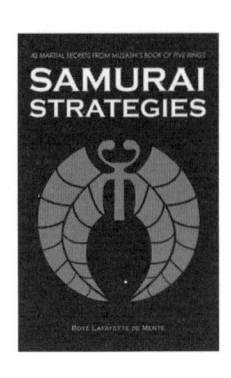

SAMURAI STRATEGIES
42 Martial Secrets from Musashi's Book of Five Rings
by Boyé Lafayette De Mente
5 ¼ X 8, 128 pp., Paperback, $12.95
ISBN-10: 0-8048-3683-3
ISBN-13: 978-0-8048-3683-8

17th-century strategies full of valuable insights for anyone in any field of endeavor—from business, war, and sports to art, love, and politics.

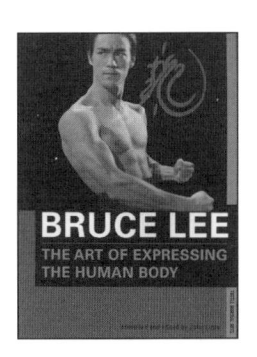

THE ART OF EXPRESSING THE HUMAN BODY
by Bruce Lee
8 ½ X 11, 256 pp., Paperback, $19.95
ISBN-10: 0-8048-3129-7
ISBN-13: 978-0-8048-3129-1

Bruce Lee's intensive and ever-evolving conditioning regime is revealed for the first time in this book.

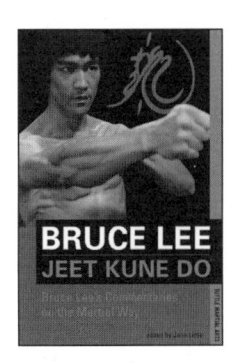

JEET KUNE DO
Bruce Lee's Commentaries on the Martial Way
by Bruce Lee
6 X 9, 400 pp., Paperback, $19.95
ISBN-10: 0-8048-3132-7
ISBN-13: 978-0-8048-3132-1

Based on never before published material by Bruce Lee, this landmark book serves as a complete presentation of the art of Jeet Kune Do.

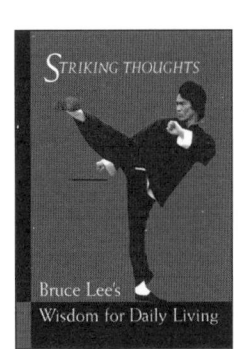

STRIKING THOUGHTS
Bruce Lee's Wisdom for Daily Living
by Bruce Lee
5 X 7 ½, 256 pp., Paperback, $12.95
ISBN-10: 0-8048-3471-7
ISBN-13: 978-0-8048-3471-1

Legendary among practitioners of martial arts, this book outlines the techniques and philosophies Lee used to develop his personal philosophy as well as the fighting system of Jeet Kune Do.

THE STRAIGHT LEAD

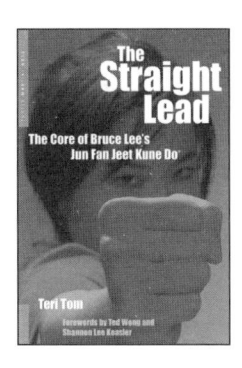

The Core of Bruce Lee's Jun Fan Jeet Kune Do®
by Teri Tom
6 ¾ X 9 ¾, 224 pp., Paperback, $19.95
ISBN-10: 0-8048-3630-2
ISBN-13: 978-0-8048-3630-2

"Presents a truly accurate perspective on the development of the straight lead, and a truly meaningful contribution to the study and appreciation of Jeet Kune Do and the man who created it, Bruce Lee." —Ted Wong

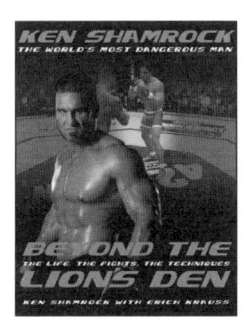

BEYOND THE LION'S DEN

The Life, the Fights, the Techniques
by Ken Shamrock with Erich Krauss
8 ½ X 11, 288 pp., Paperback, $29.95
ISBN-10: 0-8048-3659-0
ISBN-13: 978-0-8048-3659-3

"As soon as you get this book, you will automatically put everything else down. Guaranteed. There's no way you can resist checking it out." —*Grappling*

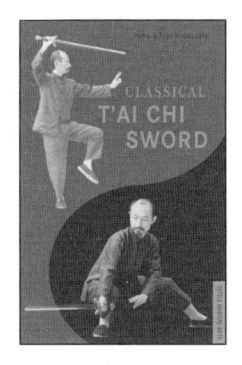

CLASSICAL T'AI CHI SWORD

by Petra and Toyo Kobayashi
6 X 9, 176 pp., Paperback, $18.95
ISBN-10: 0-8048-3448-2
ISBN-13: 978-0-8048-3448-3

In T'ai Chi Ch'uan, exercising with a sword has developed into an important art. *Classsical T'ai Chi Sword* presents a clearly illustrated introduction to the sword practice, complete with photographs, diagrams, and step-by-step instructions.

MORE TAI CHI BOOKS FROM TUTTLE PUBLISHING

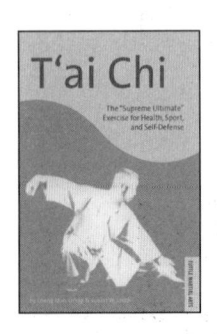

T'AI CHI
The "Supreme Ultimate" Exercise for Health, Sport, and Self-Defense
by Cheng Man-ch'ing and Robert W. Smith
6 X 9, 128 pp., Paperback, $19.95
ISBN-10: 0-8048-3593-4
ISBN-13: 978-0-8048-3593-0

This book is a complete step-by-step manual for the beginner that will enable anyone to master the T'ai-chi solo exercise.

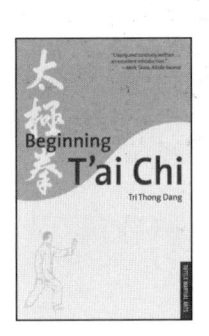

BEGINNING T'AI CHI
by Tri Thong Dang
6 X 9, 72 pp., Paperback, $10.95
ISBN-10: 0-8048-2001-5
ISBN-13: 978-0-8048-2001-1

In this handy guide, Master Tri Thong Dang, an instructor for over three decades, describes T'ai Chi's simplified form: a set of movements specifically designed for beginners. Concise descriptions highlight the spiritual essence of T'ai Chi and display its graceful simplicity.

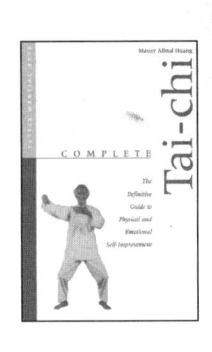

COMPLETE TAI-CHI
The Definitive Guide to Physical and Emotional Self-Improvement
by Alfred Huang
6 X 9, 280 pp., Paperback, $19.95
ISBN-10: 0-8048-1897-5
ISBN-13: 978-0-8048-1897-1

Master Huang's *Complete Tai-Chi* is the definitive introduction to the Condensed Form of Wu-style Tai-chi, a form that has gained enormous popularity as a healing exercise because it stresses the development of internal energy for self-healing.